HOW TO TALK TO YOUR DOCTOR

THE QUESTIONS TO ASK

JANET R. MAURER, M.D.

A FIRESIDE BOOK
PUBLISHED
BY
SIMON & SCHUSTER,
INC.
NEW YORK

◆

PUBLISHED BY SIMON & SCHUSTER, INC.
SIMON & SCHUSTER BUILDING
ROCKEFELLER CENTER
1230 AVENUE OF THE AMERICAS
NEW YORK, NEW YORK 10020
FIRESIDE AND COLOPHON ARE REGISTERED
TRADEMARKS OF SIMON & SCHUSTER, INC.
DESIGNED BY BONNI LEON
MANUFACTURED IN THE UNITED STATES OF AMERICA
2   4   6   8   10   9   7   5   3   1
LIBRARY OF CONGRESS CATALOGING IN
PUBLICATION DATA

Maurer, Janet R.
How to talk to your doctor.

"A Fireside book."
1. Physician and patient.   2. Patient education.
3. Consumer education.   I. Title.   [DNLM: 1. Patient
Education—popular works.   2. Physician-Patient
Relations—popular works. W 85 M453h]
R727.3.M377   1986   610.69′6   86–3802

ISBN: 0–671–60390–6

ACKNOWLEDGMENT
TO
MARILYN, WHO TYPED
AND TYPED
AND TYPED

TO MY PATIENTS

CONTENTS

◆

INTRODUCTION

◆

When I began practicing medicine, I found that many patients seemed to accept blindly whatever explanation or information I gave them about their health.

Though I was certain I must be overlooking many concerns they had, the reply I most often received to my plea "Don't you have some questions?" was a blank stare!

It was only after a particularly assertive patient eventually answered, "I do, but I don't know enough to know what to ask," that I realized *most* people do not know *what* to ask.

Most people have no idea how an illness can affect their future, family, and job. Most have no idea of the complexities of therapy or the potential for developing complications and side effects. Most do not know how to find sources to learn about disease, or what to do if they feel uncertain about their care. This book is for those people.

This is a handbook for patients. It is designed to educate them about their medical problems. It is meant to foster a cooperative effort between patients and doctors, because this is the most positive approach and the most likely to improve health care. In addition to giving you the questions you need to have answered, this book expresses my philosophy about medical care: that there is little room for adversarial relationships in medicine, that mutual education and cooperation help create the optimum environment for achieving the best level of health possible.

The book's design makes it easy to refer to questions in areas of immediate concern. There is some overlapping between chapters so that you will not have to turn continually from one chapter to another. You will find, for instance, some questions listed under specific illnesses like cancer similar to those found in the chapter on illnesses in general.

Take the book with you on your visits with your doctor. Review the pertinent questions in the waiting room. Then, if they are not answered in the course of your examination, ask them! You will feel much better informed. He will be encouraged by your interest and probably volunteer information. Chances are your relationship will benefit along with your understanding of your body and overall sense of well-being.

CHAPTER ONE

◆

THE
PATIENT-
DOCTOR
RELATIONSHIP

◆

The key to receiving the best medical care is to have a relaxed and open relationship with your doctor. Aside from feeling more comfortable, there is a very important reason for this. Your doctor should know a good deal more about you than the *facts* of your illness. Medicine is often an inexact science, and often several approaches are equally appropriate—whether it is in making a diagnosis, prescribing therapy or following up a particular problem. In deciding the approach to take in your particular case, your doctor will gauge your personality, your general philosophy about your health, your ability and desire to participate in your own care, and your ability to understand and cope with illness. In specific situations, your pain threshold, your self-image or your vanity may influence a medical decision. The two of you will establish and maintain a good rapport only if you are both completely honest and frank with each other. Otherwise, you may feel uncomfortable in asking questions and unhappy with the course of your care, because the doctor lacked information that might have led to a more appropriate approach for you.

For example, you may be terrified of any medical procedure involving a needle, but also very good at hiding this anxiety. You have recently had pneumonia and feel better, but a new chest x-ray shows abnormal fluid (a pleural effusion) around your left lung. Your doctor has decided to perform a thoracentesis, which involves placing a needle through the skin and muscle into the fluid and drawing the fluid out with a syringe. You agree to the procedure, but neglect to mention your fear of needles and successfully hide your anxiety. As the doctor takes out the tiny needle to give the local anesthetic, you can no longer control your anxiety. You feel sick to your stomach, lightheaded, and pass out. You fall off the chair, bump your head on the floor and have to be admitted to the hospital for observation. If the doctor had known about your fears, you could have been given a tranquilizer and mild sedative and the procedure would have taken a few minutes. Instead, you have a headache, a hospital bill, and a canceled thoracentesis. Both you and the doctor are frustrated. If the doctor does not make an effort to get to know you as a person, *or* if you do not allow it, building frustrations will cause resentment and a growing distance between you.

If you have traditionally thought of physicians as "godlike," it will be difficult to know what to expect from your doctor and what to contribute to the relationship. Here is an approach that may help form a more workable relationship. You are paying for a specific service. Your physician is highly trained and uniquely qualified to provide this service for you—as are many other professionals in their field. For this reason, your doctor deserves your respect. In return, you can expect a competent, professional job. That is, you can expect a thorough, careful evaluation of your symptoms and a clear discussion regarding diagnosis, treatment, and prognosis. You should participate as fully as you can by asking appropriate questions. It is not reasonable to expect cures for incurable diseases or simple, rapid evaluations and treatment of complex, serious problems. In the following pages, I will list the basic rights and responsibilities in a good patient-doctor relationship. The specifics may not be fully appropriate in every case, but they make a good general set of rules that should facilitate doctor-patient discussion and result in good rapport.

THE PATIENT'S RIGHTS

♦ 1   Have as much information as he/she wishes about the illness

You come to the physician to gain understanding of your health and you pay for this. You have the right to know your diagnosis, prognosis, alternate forms of treatment, recommendations of your doctor and why. If a diagnosis has not been reached, you should have a clear explanation of why not. Also, if further studies or follow-up is indicated, this should be explained. It is, after all, your body and your health that are in the balance.

♦ 2   Be allowed adequate time for questions and concerns about problems

To be fully informed about your illness, usually more than one appointment will be necessary. Often hearing a diagnosis takes you by surprise and you forget some information or do not think of the appropriate questions until later. Thus, you should have an opportunity both at the initial visit and at subsequent times to discuss your problems. Questions should be written down so they will be at your fingertips at the follow-up visit.

♦ 3   **Have reasonable access to the doctor**

This must be agreed upon in advance. You might feel it important to have frequent access (say, weekly appointments), but your physician may feel this is unnecessary and monthly or quarterly appointments are adequate. Possibly a compromise can be worked out. If it cannot, you should establish this early, so you can find another physician, because this kind of issue will lead to countless annoyances and difficulties in the relationship.

♦ 4   **Participate in major decisions in your care**

Participation is not only the right but also the responsibility of the patient. To do this appropriately, you must be well educated about your illness and must ask questions so your decisions—with the guidance and assistance of your doctor—are as informed as possible. You and your family are going to be the main persons affected by your illness, not your doctor, and the sooner you realize this the easier it will be to deal with the illness.

♦ 5   **Know the physician's nonoffice-hour availability and provisions for coverage of patients during those times**

You may need a physician at the least expected time. Emergencies, accidents, and crises always seem to occur during nights, weekends, and holidays. Who is available when your own doctor is not? If at all possible, you should arrange to meet the covering doctors so you can decide whether you can work with them. Remember the substitute may be your doctor during your most vulnerable and neediest times.

◆ 6   Determine who other than the doctor shall have access to information about your health

The relationship of the physician and the patient is confidential. However, the patient may make a signed request to have his files released to certain individuals, usually insurance companies, compensation boards, or other physicians. In some cases where a disease is infectious (e.g., tuberculosis) or otherwise might affect the health of others (e.g., seizures), the doctor is legally obligated to report the condition to governmental authorities.

◆ 7   Know in advance the approximate amount of charges and possible arrangements for payment

It is *not* poor taste to ask about charges in advance. You need to determine whether you can afford the services or whether insurance will cover them. Also, if you cannot afford the charges, many doctors will work out a sliding scale based on your ability to pay. Determine exactly what the charges include because some things may not be included: laboratory tests, for example. Also, check in *advance* what your insurance will cover as well as the amount of the deductible.

◆ 8   Be seen within a reasonable time of the scheduled appointment

Occasionally, unexpected issues arise in the evaluation of patients preceding you that cause delay in your appointment time. These situations are unforeseeable and cannot be helped. A half-hour wait is probably not unreasonable as long as the receptionist informs you of the delay. Some doctors are chronically late. Decide if this is an intolerable annoyance in terms of wasted time, and if so, choose a physician who is prompt, rather than being repeatedly annoyed at his tardiness.

◆ 9   Change physicians if a breakdown in your relationship occurs and have your records transferred to your new doctor

Occasionally, as in any relationship, unsolvable conflicts will arise which may destroy your confidence in or ability to work with your doctor. Do not allow this situation to persist. For more information about changing doctors in unsatisfying circumstances, see Chapter 8.

THE PATIENT'S RESPONSIBILITIES

♦ 1   **Disclose all information relating to your illness to the physician**

The doctor cannot be expected to make an accurate diagnosis and institute proper therapy if some information is withheld. In fact, withholding or misstating data requested by the doctor may result in the use of improper, even potentially dangerous therapies or risky tests. Information you give your doctor is confidential; any information you give should not be used in any way other than to better direct your care. Often, information relating to your illness will include information about your family, home and work situation, and previous medical problems, because all of these things influence one's health.

♦ 2   **Keep office appointments or cancel well in advance**

Just as it is unfair for the doctor to make you wait excessively, it is unfair for you not to keep appointments. If you expect to be late, call and let the receptionist know. If you are not going to use scheduled time, someone else should be allowed to. Cancellations should be made at least 24 hours in advance.

♦ 3   **Plan your visit with the physician**

It is important to think about your complaint in advance and to organize the kinds of questions you want answered. Think carefully about your symptoms, so you can give informed answers to the doctor's questions. For example, when exactly does the pain begin? How long does it last? What relieves it? Does it wake you at night? Your meeting time will accomplish what you and the doctor want, and neither of you will be frustrated by discussion of extraneous subjects.

♦ 4   Stop the doctor when you do not understand what he is explaining and ask for a simpler explanation

How is the doctor to know when you do not understand? He will not think you are stupid if you ask for clarification; he will probably welcome your participation. Remember, it is difficult for the doctor—who is knowledgeable about your illness—to imagine himself as someone who knows very little. Yet he must do this to explain your situation adequately. He may have lapses and inadvertently assume you have a wider knowledge than you do. If this happens, gently remind him that you are not so educated.

♦ 5   Ask questions

This is as much a responsibility of the patient as it is a right. No matter how well he knows you, the physician cannot read your mind and anticipate all of your particular concerns. You must ask the appropriate questions. See Chapters 2 and 3 for help in finding those that apply to you.

♦ 6   Follow physician advice and report quickly any adverse effects of therapy, complications from tests, or worsening symptoms

Nothing is quite as annoying to a doctor as a patient who won't follow instructions. Why did you come in the first place? This is noncompliance. Now, if there is some legitimate reason for this, the doctor should be informed so appropriate changes can be made. He cannot be expected to be on top of your problems if you don't keep him informed.

♦ 7   Limit intervisit phone calls to the problems listed in 6 above or other agreed-upon matters

While it is important to inform the doctor of the problems noted above, it is equally important not to "bug" him.

The doctor may ask you to call for test results and, of course, you should report changes in your condition. Often, doctors will wait several hours to return nonemergency calls so as not to interrupt ward rounds, patient visits, and so on. Don't be impatient if the secretary has taken a message; the doctor will get it and return your call.

♦ 8   **Pay agreed-upon charges promptly or in a way mutually acceptable to both parties**

Again, remember you are obtaining a service from your doctor just as you might from any other professional. He has a right to expect payment from you or your insurance for professional handling of your case, even if you aren't "cured." Make arrangements for payment before your visit. Illnesses often cannot be cured, only treated, and if the response to treatment is less than expected, many factors may be involved; it should not be taken out on the physician through failure to pay him.

THE PHYSICIAN'S RIGHTS

♦ 1   **Full disclosure by the patient of all data pertinent to the presenting complaints**

Only with full information can the physician request certain tests, make a diagnosis, and recommend treatment in an intelligent and informed way. Obviously, it is in your best interest to have the most correct and informed care, because it is your health that is at stake. All information you give is confidential, as stated earlier, unless you give permission for it to be disclosed *or* you have a condition that requires legal disclosures.

♦ 2   **Have adequate time for a full patient evaluation and necessary tests before making a diagnosis or starting therapy**

When you call to arrange an appointment, the doctor will probably be booked at least several days in advance. You will be scheduled at a time when a full evaluation can be done. It is unfair to yourself and the other scheduled patients to demand to be seen sooner, since both of you will be allotted much less time. Of course, if you have severe pain or similar symptoms, say so, and you will be seen as an emergency. Tests or follow-up visits may be scheduled up to a few weeks in advance. Be patient in the meantime. Very few illnesses change appreciably over a day or even weeks. Before the test results are in, the doctor may not have enough information to make a diagnosis or start therapy: it takes time to receive test reports. Again, if the doctor feels you have an emergent illness, he will either see you sooner or arrange for your evaluation by someone else. If you are unhappy with the arrangements that are made, ask for another referral.

♦ 3   **Prompt notification of worsening or change in symptoms, reactions to medications, or other health-related items**

Since everyone is unique, manifestations of any illness or response to treatment may also be unique. It is often impossible for the doctor to predict in advance any adverse side effects of drugs or directions the illness decides to take. Thus, to ensure continued appropriate management and the best therapy for you, you must maintain a good line of communication with the doctor.

♦ 4   **Act professionally in the best interest of the patient**

Occasionally, what the patient wants and what the doctor thinks is in the patient's best interest are different. There should be no broaching the rules of the relationship, e.g., confidentiality; don't expect the doctor to do something that is morally repugnant to him, professionally compromising, illegal, or which he feels may harm you. If such a conflict arises, it is usually best for the doctor to withdraw from your care or alternately for you to find another doctor with whom you can work more effectively.

♦ 5   **Withdraw from the care of a patient with whom a personality conflict or emotional involvement exists or who refuses to follow his recommendations**

Physicians may experience feelings of anger or other unresolvable personality conflicts with patients. Or a doctor may find that he is developing too much emotional involvement with a patient and feel he cannot deliver care objectively. Noncompliance by a patient may also cause feelings of frustration and anger which may make it impossible to deliver good care.

The physician has the same rights as the patient to end an unsatisfactory relationship which no longer serves either party. If, however, the physician decides to sever a relationship, he should offer to arrange for continuing care by another physician for urgent problems, at least temporarily, and make available the medical records.

◆ 6   Efficient use of time

Doctors schedule patients closely and often are heavily booked. Just as you would expect someone visiting you for a specific reason to come prepared, you should organize your thoughts, think about the specifics of your symptoms, and carefully write down your questions about your problem. Not only does this make time spent with the doctor more efficient, your thoughts and questions are also organized, and you are more likely to gain a better understanding of your illness. You will remember more of what the doctor tells you and will make fewer phone calls between visits for clarification.

◆ 7   Receive prompt payment for services

Nothing can destroy a relationship as quickly as hassles over money. You should obtain information in advance about the projected fees; once you know the charges and have decided to use the services of the doctor, you have the same obligation as you would at the grocery store to pay promptly. The physician, in turn, has bills to pay. Often physicians will adjust fees according to the person's ability to pay and will also assist in filing (or actually submit) insurance claims for you.

◆ 8   Be free from patient responsibility when not in the office or on call

The doctor has a personal life. When he is not in the office or on call, he is off duty and you should respect that. It is unfair to expect the doctor to be available for you at night, on weekends, and at other private times. To calm your fears about his covering physicians when he is not available, ask to meet and talk with them. Your medical records should be available to the covering physicians if you have an emergent problem.

PHYSICIAN RESPONSIBILITIES

◆ 1   **Discuss thoroughly with the patient in nontechnical terms the diagnosis(es), work-up, therapy, and prognosis**

Probably the most common failing of physicians is to explain health problems and the related issues thoroughly and repeatedly to the patient. First, the doctor may be so familiar with the illness that he doesn't realize he is skipping vital basic information. Sometimes, you may find you have to do the reminding. Second, the doctor may feel you do not want a lot of information; if so, ask questions or simply say, "I need more information to understand and cope with my rheumatoid arthritis." Third, some doctors believe that patients "can't handle" the technical information or whole truth about their problems. Such an antiquated approach has little room in modern medical practice.

Remember, the doctor's responsibility is to the patient (if he is an adult), and as such it is inappropriate for other family members—children, parents, siblings— to ask the doctor not to discuss the illness with the person affected. It is the patient's health that is at stake, and it should be only his decision if he does not wish information.

◆ 2   **Present to the patient, when appropriate, alternative generally accepted approaches to therapy or to reaching a diagnosis even if the physician does not personally accept them**

There are often several approaches to therapy or to establishing a diagnosis. These will vary some among physicians, institutions, or even parts of the country depending on philosophies, availability of sophisticated medical testing and therapeutic equipment, and regional successes with therapy. For example, if you have certain types of coronary artery disease with pain (angina pectoris), some doctors would recommend heart surgery (which now has a death risk of less than 5%), whereas others would recommend medication (which has some potential side effects). Neither may be better in terms of survival. With surgery there is the risk of death; with drugs the prospect is lifelong medication with some potential side effects. You should be aware of both approaches; one may be more acceptable because of fear of surgery, expense, inconvenience, self-image, or other personal reasons. The physician should present to you the relative pros and cons of each approach and then follow guideline number 3 next.

◆ 3 Recommend to the patient what the physician considers the best approach and explain why

While it is important for your doctor to make you aware of alternative approaches, it is just as important for him to recommend what he feels is best for you. To some extent, these recommendations reflect his bias, but they also take into account other factors which are peculiar to you. He will, in recommending therapy, consider the disease as it is present in you (e.g., it may take a very mild form and therefore, be most amenable to observation only), your personality, your approach to illness, your ability to comply with recommended treatment, your work demands, your family supports, or whatever unique factors exist in your case.

If after this has all been explained to you, you are still uncertain whether you want to proceed with therapy, you must inform the doctor. Either the two of you will be able to agree on an alternative, or if not, he can refer you to another physician.

◆ 4 Allow adequate time (on at least one additional occasion) to answer patient questions and discuss patient concerns

Often the initial visit to the doctor is sort of a blur. You may be nervous and you will not remember much information. Questions will not occur to you until you walk out the door. Thus, it is critical for you to have time to adjust emotionally to a new diagnosis or treatment. As this occurs, you will find yourself with more unanswered questions. Thus, at least a second session, if only for talking to the doctor or counseling, is really necessary. This is also a good way of making sure medications are taken correctly. The doctor's failure to allow for, or the patient's failure to take advantage of, this second session can be a major factor in a breakdown of the relationship. It can also lead to misconceptions about the illness, misunderstanding about medication regimens, and other problems.

♦ 5 **Provide adequate follow-up and emergency care and make patients aware of this**

Providing quality care to patients includes making clear-cut arrangements for handling of emergent problems or problems that occur during nonoffice hours. Though doctors usually have busy office schedules, they will often keep one or two appointment slots open for patients with emergent problems. If this option is not available, the doctor should either provide for emergency-room care for the patient or arrange with another doctor to see overflow patients. Also, each doctor should have an arrangement (which is readily available and easily understood) for weekend, holiday, and night coverage. If patients wish, the physician should make provisions for them to meet the covering doctor before emergencies occur.

♦ 6 **Ask for specialist consultation or a second opinion when uncertain about a diagnosis**

Every physician has had the experience of being stumped. So much new information is generated through medical research each year that it is impossible for the internist to keep up on all diseases. Most doctors realize that occasionally they will encounter difficulties in diagnosis or treating a particular patient. The same illness never looks quite the same in different people. Sometimes the doctor simply cannot be sure with which illness he is dealing. At this point the internist should arrange for a visit to a doctor whose specialty likely includes the disease in question. For example, a person with inflamed joints might be sent to a rheumatologist. The primary care of the patient lies with his internist, however, and generally this specialist will simply make recommendations for the primary doctor to carry out.

◆ 7   **Assist in obtaining relevant social services or rehabilitation services for the patient**

The total care of the patient, especially in chronic illness, extends far beyond the specific treatment of the disease. Patients may need to obtain special facilities for their homes, e.g., wheelchairs, or may need an in-home housekeeper or nursing service because of their illness. Rehabilitation of patients with paralysis, chronic lung disease, heart, kidney, and many other illnesses may be a critical part of the care. Your doctor or his staff should be able to refer you to the appropriate agencies and assist you in obtaining these ancillary services. Other problems may occur within the family that require psychological or psychiatric intervention. Appropriate referral for these services should also be available.

◆ 8   **Keep complete patient records**

It is both a legal and moral obligation of a physician to keep complete care records of his patients. This assures a smooth transition, for whatever reason, of care from one physician to another. It also helps prevent unfortunate errors because memory fails on exact medication doses or on exactly what was decided at what visit or during what phone conversation. Finally, it is crucial as documentation in any legal proceeding brought for whatever reason.

◆ 9   **Assist in a smooth transition for the patient to another doctor when a relationship has been ended**

If, for whatever reason, your care has been transferred to another doctor, your former doctor should facilitate the move by promptly forwarding records (at your written request), and if necessary discussing your case with the new doctor. This is true also in situations where the change in doctors is caused by your or his moving to a new location.

◆ **10   Make available to patients a list of his charges for the services he performs**

All physicians have some system for charging their patients. Often, initial visits are one charge, follow-up visits a somewhat lesser charge. The doctor should have available a summary of his usual charges so you will know what sort of financial commitment you are making when you visit him. Often, doctors will reduce fees for patients who are not able to pay the full charge. Also remember that physician fees do not pay for laboratory tests or the services of other persons or equipment that may be needed.

These guidelines should give you a feeling for what can reasonably be expected from your doctor and what you should contribute. They do not establish the relationship. That takes effort from both of you. Good relationships, remember, need to be nurtured, so maintain openness and frank discussion throughout your relationship with your doctor.

CHAPTER TWO

◆

UNDERSTANDING
YOUR ILLNESS

◆

We all dread becoming ill. Even something as simple as a cold brings discomfort and disrupts our daily routines. Worse yet, the disease itself can be very frightening either because of its seriousness or, more often, because we do not know how serious it is. The best way to get the information that will allay these fears is to ask questions. The better educated we are, the easier it is to cope with and overcome any illness. This chapter will help you organize your thoughts so you can ask your doctor important and relevant questions.

As a first step, let us take a look at how the physician puts together the pieces of information you give him to arrive at a specific diagnosis or to narrow the possible diagnoses.

Because our bodies are so complex, many of the parts may malfunction in a variety of ways: they can break, wear out, be attacked by hostile bacteria or by our own immune systems, or become cancerous. If any of these malfunctions interfere with the body's normal performance, they may be experienced as symptoms of disease.

The physician's role is first to ascertain the most likely site of a malfunction, second to find the cause, and finally to correct the problem if possible. If it cannot be corrected, he will try to alleviate the symptoms.

He begins by obtaining from you a detailed *history* of your symptoms. The history is the most crucial step in reaching a correct diagnosis. It alerts the doctor to look for certain things during the physical examination and to order certain laboratory tests. During the history the doctor will ask about other things besides your symptoms. Questions about previous medical and surgical problems, family diseases, allergies, habits, hobbies, work history, places you have traveled, any other ongoing medical problems, and what medications you take all help to put your symptoms in perspective and give a better insight into your general health.

These questions will be quite detailed. It is not enough to know that you have a pain in your stomach. It is necessary to know if the pain is in the upper or lower abdomen; if it is sharp, dull, achy, burning; if it is fleeting or lasts for minutes or hours; if it is constant or intermittent; if it occurs in the morning or evening;

if it occurs with meals or before or after meals; if it is relieved or worsened or unchanged by eating; and so on. Only by eliciting this type of detail will your doctor be able to pinpoint the organ system from which the symptoms most likely come and what might be the cause. This type of questioning may seem endless, especially when you do not feel well, but always remember that your accurate and complete answers are essential to making a correct diagnosis.

Next is the physical examination. Generally, the doctor will start by examining your head and neck and work toward your lower limbs. However, following the leads you have given in the history, he will be looking for certain specific physical findings and will probably spend the most time examining those areas where you are complaining of symptoms. You will usually be asked to take off your clothes and put on a loose-fitting gown for the exam. The doctor will uncover only the part of the body he is examining and then recover that part when he moves on to another area. He will respect your modesty as much as possible, but he must be able to see the area he is examining to do an accurate evaluation.

Normally, the physical is not painful. If during the exam you feel pain or discomfort be sure to mention the troublesome area to the doctor because he might not be aware of a problem there. When he is finished, if you feel the doctor has overlooked something—like a change in a mole which might not be obvious—mention it. Do not assume it has been seen; doctors miss things too. In fact, if you are concerned about anything, make it a special point to ask. Even if it turns out to be nothing, you at least will not worry unnecessarily.

One further point to keep in mind is that you have a right to expect certain evaluations to be done as routine during a physical examination. Women should have pelvic examinations and Pap smears done and a thorough breast examination no matter what their age. All persons over 40 should have rectal examinations, checking of the stool for blood, and testing of the eyes for glaucoma. These evaluations are designed to pick up early disease that can be successfully treated.

The final segment of the "work-up" is the laboratory evaluation. Sometimes a problem is simple to diagnose and no laboratory tests are needed. Other times they may be done either to aid in making the diagnosis, to confirm the diagnosis, or to follow the response to therapy. Often, especially in patients over age 40, a routine set of blood tests will be ordered. These are done to establish the usual, or baseline, values of certain chemical components in your blood and the red and white blood cell counts. Besides establishing baseline values these same tests can be used to screen for certain diseases, e.g., kidney disease and diabetes (high blood sugar). Other commonly ordered tests which are used to screen for common illnesses are urine analysis (urinalysis), chest x-ray, and a tracing of the heart's electrical activity (electrocardiogram, ECG). In women over 40, a mammogram is recommended by many as a screening test for breast cancer. (Please refer to Chapter 5 for more discussion of laboratory tests.) If the history and/or physical suggest a specific illness or organ involvement, specialized tests to check on that specific problem will probably be done.

Keep in mind, however, that the laboratory work is usually merely supporting evidence for a diagnosis or helps to rule out an alternate possibility. More than 90 percent of the time, the doctor will be reasonably certain of the diagnosis by the end of the history and physical.

Now how can all that information be fit together to arrive at the diagnosis? Though there are many ways of organizing the data, here are two common and complementary steps that many physicians use. You can get a feel for how complex the process is.

First, the doctor will try to identify the *organ system* involved. For example, if the pain is located in the chest he will have tried to characterize the pain, because pressing pain is more often angina (the heart), burning pain more often heartburn (the gut), knifelike pain that increases with deep breaths more often pleural (the lining around the lungs), and achy and dull pain more often chest wall (muscles). Or do the symptoms seem to involve more than one area and therefore more than one organ system, which might imply a generalized disorder?

Once the organ system(s) involved is identified, the second step is to establish the *cause* of the symptoms. This is nearly always necessary before a definite diagnosis can be made and therapy started.

Often the story that you have told to the physician and what he has found on the physical exam are similar to other cases he has seen or read about, and he will recognize a certain type of illness. However, diseases almost never have the same symptoms or all of the symptoms expected from "classic" descriptions because each person is different and responds to illness in different ways. Thus, it is not uncommon for you and your neighbor who have the same illness to have quite different sets of complaints. Sometimes, these variations on a theme may suggest other less likely but possible diagnoses—called a differential diagnosis—and laboratory tests will be ordered in an attempt to pin down the final diagnosis more positively.

The more common types, categories, or causes of disease the physician may be thinking about while trying to work out the diagnosis include the following:

AUTOIMMUNE: When the body forms antibodies (proteins directed against foreign substances) to oppose some of its own tissues, resulting in malfunction or destruction of organs, this is called autoimmune disease. Complexes of antigens (substances perceived as foreign by one's body) and antibodies might deposit in specific tissues causing the disease in those tissues; antibodies to one's tissues might directly attach to the organs perceived as foreign; or the major symptoms and destruction might come from inflammation that is stimulated by the antibody formation. With modern technology many diseases whose cause was previously unknown have been found to be caused by autoantibodies. A sampling of autoimmune diseases includes systemic lupus erythematosus, rheumatoid arthritis, and some thyroid diseases.

CONGENITAL: Diseases present at birth as a result of either heredity or a mishap in development of the fetus are congenital. The signs of the illness or developmental malformation may or may not be apparent, however. Some diseases in this group are not obvious until adulthood, like Huntington's chorea, a disease of the nervous system in which movement disorders occur and, eventually, senility. Another example is retinitis pigmentosa, a disease that results in blindness.

DEGENERATIVE: Degenerative refers simply to diseases resulting from body parts wearing out. These, of course, become more common with age. Included here are some forms of arthritis and some heart valve diseases, for example.

IDIOPATHIC: When the cause of a disease is uncertain, it is placed in this category.

INFECTIOUS: Illnesses caused by microorganisms invading and multiplying in body tissues are called infections. The body's reaction to these invaders is inflammation (see below), but often the symptoms, e.g. fever, are caused by the organisms themselves. Infections at one time were a major cause of death, especially in children and young adults, but the twentieth-century development of multiple antibiotics has made cures often possible in this category of illness.

INFLAMMATORY: This is a broad range of illnesses in which the body's immune system, a system composed of white blood cells and other factors that defend the body against bacteria and other foreign materials, plays a primary role. This might be an appropriate defensive role when the body is infected by disease-causing organisms, or there might be an inappropriate overresponse, as when a hypersensitivity (allergic) reaction occurs. Or there might be an actual derangement of the system, as in the autoimmune diseases (discussed previously), when the tissue-destructive properties of the inflammatory cells are directed against the normal body cells.

NEOPLASTIC: Neoplastic literally means "new thing formed" or "new growth." People often interpret neoplasm as cancer, which is an uncontrolled growth of abnormal cells. This, however, represents only one type of neoplastic disease. Many neoplasms are *benign* rather than malignant. That is, while new growth of cells occurs and is abnormal in that area, it is not uncontrolled growth and generally will not spread and cause death. Noncancerous neoplasms include uterine fibroids, lipomas, and hamartomas, for example.

TRAUMATIC: Injury to the body from a source outside the body is called trauma. Traumatic disease might include a broken arm from a car accident, a ruptured spleen from a fall while skiing, or a collapsed lung from broken ribs sustained in a fall from a roof.

VASCULAR: This group of diseases overlaps somewhat with several other categories in that some of the diseases that occur in vessels are caused by inflammatory cells, degenerative changes, and so on. Yet there are a large number of diseases in vessels that are not really in these groups and that are not really included elsewhere. I prefer to separate them from the other groups. Some physicians do not. Examples include narrowing of vessels that results in high pressures in the vessels or the tendency to form clots and the sequelae of that clot formation.

MISCELLANEOUS: I would place here those diseases that are not themselves inflammatory, degenerative, etc., but are from another process that is. Impaired mental function caused by a derangement of blood chemistry is an example. The patient may have some other disease process, but the mental impairment comes from the chemical abnormality.

Other illnesses in this category might include those caused by the effects of drugs ingested either to treat other diseases or for recreation or in suicide attempts.

Some physicians rearrange these categories and separate out large subcategories, e.g., metabolic disease, as I did for vascular disease. But regardless of how the outline is arranged, the approach is similar. Now that you have an understanding of how your doctor might organize and distill the information you give him, let us look at how *you* can get the information you want from him.

BASIC PRINCIPLES

When you ask questions about your health, you will find the answers more satisfying and your thoughts better focused if you follow these general principles:

1. Make clear that you are interested in learning about your general health or illness. Some patients do not wish to know much about their illnesses and physicians are sensitive to that. But if you make a simple introductory statement like "I'd really like to learn more about this problem," your doctor will be much more likely to take the time to explain in detail and to answer questions.

2. Volunteer facts you feel might have been overlooked. If after your interview, examination, and laboratory work have been done you feel something has been left out or overlooked, do not assume it is irrelevant. Always mention or ask about those things that concern you. Even if it is not important, no harm is done by mentioning it, and you will have peace of mind.

3. Make your questions specific. You are concerned about those aspects of your health that will apply to your specific life-style, job, etc. Many diseases vary in their manifestations depending on such things as your age, race, or sex. You will get more useful information about your ability to continue your favorite sport of long-distance running, for instance, not by asking, "How much exercise can I do," when what you want to know is, "Can I still run my usual ten miles a day?" You can decide how specific you will need to be by gauging the answers to the first few questions. Also, generally, the better the doctor knows you, the easier it is to anticipate your questions.

4. Conquer your fear of the unknown. All of us, when we discover something amiss with our body, be it a new pain or a lump in the breast, grasp the hope that if we ignore it, it will go away. We fear it might be something horrible. Sometimes this works and the problem disappears. But when the abnormality persists or worsens, this course becomes irrational; waiting longer to have it evaluated can only result in more serious illness. The truth is often less sinister than what you expect. Even if the news is bad, you will be much better able to cope psychologically with the disease once you hear and deal with the diagnosis. And early disease is usually much easier to treat.

5. Ask for clarification. Whenever you do not under-

stand what your doctor is saying or what it means to you, or if the statements are too general, stop him. Ask politely for picture explanations, words spelled out, simpler vocabulary, or relevance to your case. Ask to have the diagnosis and any instructions written down. Anxiety in the office makes it difficult to remember all of what is said.

6. Ask for repeat explanations. On subsequent visits, ask for a simple reexplanation of the illness or, alternatively, reserve the more in-depth questions for the second or later visits. It sometimes takes quite a while to absorb information, and often we selectively forget upsetting things like an unpleasant diagnosis or prognosis. While selective memory may be useful in helping you cope initially, it can hamper treatment and recovery.

7. Take notes. Taking notes will help you not only to remember but also to more accurately describe pertinent details about your illness to family members. This will also help you organize your thoughts to ask your doctor unanswered questions on return visits.

8. Proceed in an organized way. Try to ask all the questions about a certain aspect of the disease and then move on to another aspect. For example, if you ask how the disease is transmitted from person to person, it is logical to follow with a question about how to limit spread of the disease. If, on the other hand, you ask the first question, then intersperse a question about medication before asking the second question, your whole train of thought will be interrupted and you will be less likely to retain the information. It is also less confusing for the doctor to follow an organized approach. He is likely to give more information if the questions follow a logical sequence.

9. Be careful with statistics. You will be tempted to ask for statistics about your illness. You may want to know how many patients are cured, how effective certain medications are, how often complications develop, what your chances of living a normal life-span are. Statistics are often available to answer these questions. However, remember that statistics are derived from large groups of persons with the same disease or who have taken the same medication or who have de-

veloped the same complications, or whatever. These numbers are only helpful in giving some perspective and should be looked at that way. If you are told only 10 percent do achieve a cure, you may be very depressed. *But* 10 percent *do* achieve a cure, and if you fall into that 10 percent, the other 90 percent do not matter much, do they?

On the other hand, there are instances in which a small percentage in statistics can be given too much weight. Let's say you have a form of arthritis that is often helped by a certain pain medication, but that pain medication has a one percent chance of causing severe destruction of the bone marrow. Once you have checked to see if other medications that are less risky are available and have found they are not, you will have to weigh the benefits of relief from the arthritis pain versus the risk. A risk of one percent, even if life-threatening, may be worth it if it will significantly improve your quality of life.

10. Do not ask questions that have no answers. When you are told you have a serious illness or an incurable illness, you will probably want to know how long you can expect to live. While it is normal for you to ask about your chances of an early death, do not be surprised if your doctor seems somewhat uncomfortable with this type of question. Of course he cannot know how long you have to live or whether you will get a certain side effect from a drug or develop complications from your illness. He can only give you statistics; trying to get a precise answer may be frustrating.

THE QUESTIONS TO ASK

The answers to the following list of questions are meant to guide you to an overall understanding of your medical problems. Once you have begun the conversation, you may find that other questions arise or that some of the subsequent questions are no longer appropriate. When this is the case, adjust your approach to the situation and keep in mind the general principles outlined above. To ensure an orderly approach, questions are arranged according to these subgroups: (1)

certainty of diagnosis, (2) cause and nature of disease, (3) course of the disease, (4) treatment, and (5) implications for family, social and work life.

CERTAINTY OF DIAGNOSIS

◆ 1 Is there a possibility the diagnosis is incorrect?

Often the possible diagnoses have been narrowed to one or two, with one being much more likely, but not 100 percent certain. This may not have been made clear to you. On the other hand, the diagnosis may be certain. If the answer is no, ask the follow-up question:

◆ 2 Is any other confirmatory evaluation available and/or indicated?

More tests may be available to assess your symptoms and your physician may choose to forego them because he feels quite sure of the diagnosis or the tests pose some risk or the tests are costly and unlikely to add information. This may be the most prudent approach. However, you should have the option of knowing why this approach has been taken and be allowed to participate in the decision. If you do not feel comfortable with this, you may wish to get a second opinion.

CAUSE AND NATURE OF THE ILLNESS

◆ 1 What organs of my body are involved and in what way?

This helps you "locate" the illness. Ask for drawings and down-to-earth terms to explain the illness. Make sure you understand whether it is a growth or malfunction or whatever is involved in the illness. Do not be satisfied until you have a mental image of the nature of the problem.

◆ 2 How did I get this illness?

Make sure you use the name of the disease in asking this and future questions. This will get you familiar with the proper pronunciation of the word(s). To gain some insight into the illness, ask, "How common is this illness in my sex, age, and racial group?"

It is very important to know the possibility of transmission of the illness. If an infectious agent is involved, can it be passed to another person? If it is genetically determined, can it be inherited or was it simply an accident of nature? If your life-style or occupation caused the illness, that also is important to know so changes can be made. Remember that if the answers you are getting do not seem specific enough, change the tone of the conversation with a question like "Is it likely my work as a keypunch operator helped to cause this arthritis?" Other important follow-up questions are next.

♦ 3   **What is the chance my children will inherit this illness or a tendency toward it?**

Inheritance of genetic characteristics occurs in a number of ways. Thus in some cases children might have a 50 percent chance of inheriting a condition, in others 25 percent or less; in others only one sex may inherit illness. In still other diseases only the tendency toward a disease may be inherited, and changing the potential victim's environment, life-style, diet, etc., may prevent the illness. Make sure this is clarified.

♦ 4   **What are the chances other persons will get this illness from me?**

This question applies only to infectious diseases. If you have an infectious illness, it is important to be entirely clear on this point because some infections are not transmitted from person to person, e.g., urine infections. Others are transmitted readily, but only in the appropriate setting, e.g., venereal disease. Still others are easily spread through the air, e.g., chickenpox or tuberculosis, or through various body fluids and secretions, e.g., some forms of hepatitis. It is critical to determine the likelihood of others contracting your disease, and if this seems a possibility to ask, "What are the measures that I should take to prevent infecting others?"

COURSE OF THE DISEASE

♦ 1   Is this disease limited to the organs that are involved now, or will it progress to others?

Many illnesses begin in only one organ. However, if they are chronic diseases, they may through time extend to other organs or have secondary effects on other organ systems. Sometimes these effects, rather than the original disease, will be more life-threatening or more adversely affect one's life-style.

♦ 2   Will there be progressive damage in the organs that are currently involved?

This question should give you a good indication of the seriousness of the illness. In general, progressive damage will result in organ failure. Progressive diseases, including those that eventually involve multiple organs, often are more likely to have associated complications and are more ominous. If you have this type of disease, be sure to ask, "Since progression is likely, what is the usual time course over which this occurs?" If it takes twenty years for the complications of a disease to develop, it is likely to be a less catastrophic disease than one that runs its course in two years.

♦ 3   What complications am I at risk for and at what stage of the disease?

In certain illness, e.g., diabetes mellitus, the long-term complications are of as great a concern as the disease itself and may significantly alter a person's ability to do certain types of work and pursue certain life-styles. While in any particular person the specific complications cannot be predicted, you will want to discuss potential complications. Ask this question even if you have known someone who has had your illness, because the complications you are at risk for may be different. Potential for complications or progression of a disease often depends, among other things, on sex, age at which the disease was acquired, other illness the patient has, ability to tolerate medication, and how well the patient takes care of himself.

♦ 4   What symptoms or change in symptoms should I be concerned about?

You will need to gain some perspective on your illness. Especially when your illness is first diagnosed, it is easy to become obsessed with every little change in symptoms. Though this reaction is normal, it can drive both you and your doctor to distraction. A careful enumeration of those symptoms that should be investigated more thoroughly will give you some peace of mind. Also, if you have an appreciation for the symptoms that the disease often entails, e.g., morning stiffness in rheumatoid arthritis, you will be emotionally better equipped to cope with them.

♦ 5   Should I alert persons around me to watch for any symptoms of which I might not be aware?

In a few illnesses—such as an impending seizure or a low blood sugar reaction in diabetes mellitus—the patient may not be aware of a potentially harmful symptom or situation. If the patient with low blood sugar from too much insulin does not receive sugar, he may go into a coma or suffer seizures and possible brain damage.

♦ 6   Are there any organizations that can provide more information about my illness or help with the problems that result from my disease?

Nearly every chronic illness now has a national organization of families and victims of the disease. Also, certain medical centers are often known for their work with a specific disease and have compiled sources of information about these diseases. These organizations and centers will also be aware of any new or experimental therapies. Write down the name and address of any organization or information source; much of what your doctor says you may forget because of the stress of the moment. Getting literature about your illness will help you confront it, clarify your thoughts, and formulate other questions you want to ask. See the appendix for the addresses of some commonly sought organizations.

TREATMENT

♦ 1 **What medications are available to control the disease?**

Clarify the role of medication in your situation. In two persons with the same condition, medication may be useful in one and not the other. The potential benefits may or may not outweigh the risks, and your risks may differ from someone else's. Also, several different types of medication may be available for treatment of one disease, as asthma or angina pectoris (heart pain). Sometimes, one medication will work better than another, or combinations will be the most useful.

♦ 2 **What are the risks and the benefits of taking this medication at this point in my illness?**

All drugs have some side effects and therefore risk to taking them. Occasionally, these are serious and intolerable. Alternatively, medication may be necessary to cure (e.g., antibiotics) or control (e.g., high blood pressure) the illness, thereby preventing deadly complications from the disease. You should have an active role in weighing the alternatives and deciding on medication in your particular situation.

♦ 3 **If I am unable to tolerate this medication or if it is ineffective, are alternative therapies available?**

Go through the same analysis with alternative therapies, drug or otherwise. Determine why these are not the first drugs or therapies tried—e.g., less effective, more side effects or whatever. Remember, always take notes. Write down names of drugs, dosages, side effects to be aware of, and any other pertinent information. Often, the label on the medication does not contain all the things you need to know. Please refer to Chapter 4 for more information about medications.

♦ 4 **Will I need to be hospitalized to start medication?**

Some situations require close observation when medications are started, either for appropriate adjustment of the medication to the person's illness (as in the initiation of insulin therapy for diabetes mellitus or in some cases of high blood pressure control) or because of potentially serious side effects (as in the administration of cancer chemotherapy). Find out if this adjustment period applies to you, and if so, how long you can expect to be in the hospital and if your insurance covers the hospitalization. If you need to be hospitalized for further diagnostic studies, often the treatment can be initiated during the same hospital stay.

♦ 5   How will I know if I am responding to treatment and how long will I need treatment?

Response to treatment may be a decrease in or elimination of symptoms or it may not be that easy to assess. Patients with high blood pressure can tell if they are responding adequately only if someone takes their blood pressure; diabetics only if they measure urine or blood sugar. Some illnesses require as little as one dose of medication; others may require lifelong therapy.

♦ 6   Is surgery an alternative in this illness? Would you or when would you recommend it?

Surgery has a role in many diseases, though often not as an early treatment. However, it may be curative, as in the removal of a very inflamed gallbladder. It may be a way to lessen the hardship of the long-term effects of an illness, as in the correction of misshapen joints in rheumatoid arthritis or the replacement of these joints by synthetic ones. Frequently your internist will work closely with one or two surgeons in each surgical specialty whom he or she has grown to trust. You are not obligated to use these surgeons, however, despite your internist's recommendations, if you prefer someone else.

♦ 7   Are there diet changes or other measures I can take to lessen the effects of the disease?

Increasingly, one's diet and physical conditioning are being emphasized in illness and health. Many steps that generally improve your health may have a specific impact on certain diseases. These include stopping smoking, decreasing alcohol intake, and increasing exercise. In addition, often specific changes can be made by a very motivated person which will reduce symptoms. Reducing consumption of chocolate, for example, may improve symptoms of heartburn or removing a dog or cat from your home may lessen your attacks of asthma. Specific and regularly pursued physical therapy or exercises or hot baths may improve the disability of certain types of arthritis.

♦ 8   How frequently do I need to be seen by a doctor?

Knowing in advance how often you will need to have follow-up medical care will allow you to plan for the necessary absences from work or daily routine. Frequency of follow-up care reflects not only the seriousness of the illness but the philosophy of your doctor. Thus, if you know someone with the same illness who is being followed more or less often it does not necessarily mean you are more or less seriously ill. Also, if a good deal of time is required for office appointments, you might ask if your doctor keeps weekend or evening hours. Many do.

♦ 9   How do I contact you in an emergency?

Sometimes your crisis comes when your physician is not in his office or is otherwise not available. Ask to meet those who oversee his practice when he is not there and make sure you feel comfortable with them. They may be the persons caring for you in an emergency. It is common practice for several doctors in the same specialities to cover for each other in the evening and on weekends.

♦ 10   Can I do any home monitoring of my illness that might reduce the need for office visits?

Concerned and motivated patients can easily be taught to take their own blood pressure, monitor blood and urine sugar levels, check the functioning of a heart pacemaker, and even do certain types of kidney dialysis at home. Many of these things when done at home will not only help you understand your illness better, but give you a larger role in controlling it while you reduce overall cost and time lost from work.

INFLUENCE ON FAMILY, SOCIAL, AND WORK LIFE

◆ 1 Will I be able to continue my job as a
_____?

At some time before retirement age, can this illness cause me to be unable to do this work?

This question needs to be answered early in your illness. You need to be able to plan ahead now. In some cases, the doctor will not be able to say how the disease may affect a certain livelihood. High blood pressure that is well controlled probably will not have any affect on one's job as, say, a bookkeeper. Parkinson's disease, which often results in difficulties with movement, will almost certainly interfere with one's work as an artist. You need to know if it is likely that complications that develop twenty years from now will likely impair skills. On the other hand, do not expect absolute answers here, since a disease's effects always vary from person to person. But you can get some appreciation for the outlook for groups of persons with this illness. You may wish to retrain early if it is likely the illness will cause an early retirement from your present type of work.

◆ 2 Can I expect to have to take many sick days?

If it is possible, and often it is, to know how debilitating an illness will be, it is helpful for employers and others who depend on you to know this in advance.

◆ 3 Will this illness affect my ability to obtain life or health insurance?

This is a critical question in your planning for your and your family's future. Many diagnoses of chronic disease will increase the cost of the premium; others will make it unable for you to obtain insurance. Still others, especially if medically controlled, will have no influence.

◆ **4   Ask questions about the specific hobbies, sports, family and social activities that apply to you.**
  Examples:

• Will I be able to continue raising cocker spaniels?
• Will I still be able to run three miles a day?
• Will I still be able to coach my son's Little League team?
• Will I be able to continue as president of the Jonesville Chamber of Commerce?

Before your second visit to the doctor think about those activities that are important to maintaining your life-style. Then by specific questions clarify with him those aspects of your life-style that must be altered to best accommodate your illness and protect your health. Maintain as much of your normal routine as possible, and avoid letting the illness run your and your family's lives. However, try to avoid exhaustion, and that may mean limiting some activities.

◆ **5   Should I observe any limitations on travel or on travel to certain areas?**

Rarely does travel need to be limited except to keep from becoming overtired or, e.g., in some lung diseases in which extremes of altitude may result in dangerously low blood oxygen levels. Also, if you have an illness that at any time might require sophisticated modern technology, you may be advised not to travel to areas where this technology is not available. If you plan a trip, ask the physician if there is anything in particular that might be a problem at your destination and, if you have an illness that might require emergent medical care, the name of a reliable medical facility there.

◆ **6   Will the drugs I am taking interact with alcohol or impair my ability to have sex?**

Some drugs cause nausea and vomiting when alcohol is consumed. For other drug interactions, please see Chapter 4. A number of drugs can cause impotence of varying types. Usually if this side effect occurs, other medication can be substituted, and the problem is readily reversed.

◆ **7   Will the illness or the treatment interfere with my ability to have children?**

Usually one's childbearing ability is not affected. However, there are important exceptions to this. For example, some chemotherapeutic agents used to treat cancers may cause temporary or permanent sterility. Pregnancy is ill advised while taking many drugs because of the possibility of birth defects. Pregnancy is also ill advised when a woman has certain types of illness because of the risk to the mother.

◆ **8   Will the disease or the treatment be disfiguring?**

Permanent hair loss, finger or arm deformity, skin changes, scars, or a variety of other disfigurations can result from either illness or therapy. If this is likely to occur to you, knowing about it in advance can make it much easier to cope with. Also, plastic surgery is often available to lessen the impact of the problem.

These questions should give you a good overall understanding of almost any kind of illness. In the next chapter, I have listed questions that will give you important information about eleven common types of illness. If you have one of these types, you may wish to coordinate questions from this chapter and from that section before talking to your doctor.

♦

UNDERSTANDING
SOME
COMMON
ILLNESSES

♦

Chapter 2 lists questions that should give you an adequate understanding of any illness you might have. However, in each case certain questions will be more pertinent than others. For this reason, I have selected eleven common types of illness and listed for each a series of questions upon which you should concentrate. Most of these sets of questions cover *categories* of disease, e.g., stroke, which may have any of several different causes. The questions selected for particular reference to these illnesses are meant not to preclude your asking a broader group, as suggested in Chapter 2, but to focus your inquiry. It may be best to go over Chapter 2 first, then turn to this chapter, and if the disease you are concerned about is included, read that section.

The categories included in this chapter are

1 ◆ arthritis
2 ◆ asthma
3 ◆ cancer
4 ◆ coronary artery disease
5 ◆ diabetes mellitus
6 ◆ emphysema/chronic bronchitis
7 ◆ hepatitis and/or cirrhosis of the liver
8 ◆ high blood pressure (hypertension)
9 ◆ kidney disease
10 ◆ stroke
11 ◆ ulcer disease

A R T H R I T I S

◆ 1   What kind of arthritis do I have?

Arthritis is a very general term that encompasses many diseases. It can be a disease limited to the joints (one or several joints), or part of a generalized (called systemic) disease in which joint pain and deformity are only one aspect. It is important to your understanding of how this disease may affect your life and how well it may respond to treatment to get a thorough, understandable explanation of the arthritis.

◆ 2   What is the outlook for me?

While arthritis of any kind can be very painful and potentially disabling, the systemic or inflammatory types in particular may result in rapid destruction and serious deformity of many joints. The course of these diseases is extremely variable, and your outlook in terms of disability and joint deformity, freedom from pain, etc., may be very different from that of another person with the exact same illness. You need to get a feel for where you fit into the spectrum of your specific type of arthritis.

◆ 3   How effective is the therapy, and how does it work?

Pain relief is a major factor in all arthritis therapy. Is your arthritis one for which there is only treatment for symptoms? Does the disease process continue? Do some, but not others, of the medicines or other treatments treat the *cause* of the disease? If you know what to expect, you will be able to better communicate with your doctor about how things are going and can be realistic about your expectations.

◆ 4   Will I likely need artificial joints? How successful are these joints?

It is usually only later and in more severe disease that the question of artificial joints comes up. Today technology has made excellent long-lasting artificial joints available, which can rehabilitate patients. Even though you may not be in a position at the moment to be considering artificial joints, you can find out whether this is a possible future concern and whether you should be seen by an orthopedic surgeon.

◆ 5   How often should I have blood or urine tests to monitor side effects from drugs?

Unfortunately, many of the drugs used to treat arthritis have a risk of potentially serious side effects. These most commonly include stomach irritation, rashes and effects on the bone marrow and kidney, but can include other things when more toxic drugs are needed. Most side effects can be picked up before serious damage is done by checking blood or urine tests. Whether you need this monitoring, and how often, depends on factors unique to you: the drugs you are taking, other medical problems or preexisting abnormalities, age, etc.

♦ **6   What side effects occur, and what will be the approach if they do?**

Again, the modifications in therapy that may be needed when side effects occur are highly individual. The variables include the type of side effect, how disabling or life-threatening it is, how severe your arthritis is, alternative therapies available, and other factors unique to you. The doctor, after weighing the risks, will decide to stop, will continue, or will modify doses of medications. Knowing the symptoms or signs of side effects, if any, and complying with the monitoring program will allow you to participate fully in your own care and help you to detect toxic effects of drugs early at a reversible stage.

♦ **7   Should I be doing anything special like resting or exercising the joints?**

Depending upon the type of arthritis, some doctors would recommend resting affected joints or alternately exercising joints to maintain mobility and prevent stiffness. Specific exercises for specific joints have been developed. Many doctors feel that persons with rheumatoid arthritis should rest a certain amount during the day. Other measures dealing directly with the joints and manipulation of them may be recommended.

♦ **8   Are facilities and instructions for physiotherapy available to me, and would I benefit?**

Many hospitals have outpatient physiotherapy programs. If you have certain types of arthritis or particular problems, physiotherapy may be of some value. Techniques to deal with stiffness or muscle spasms, range-of-motion exercises, special exercises for special joints, whirlpools, and so on, are some of the programs and facilities that might be available. Not all types of arthritis or types of patient are good candidates for physiotherapy, but most are.

♦ **9   Should I have any restrictions on my activity _or_ can I do anything I want?**

In some cases activity lessens stiffness and prevents muscles from atrophying (shriveling away), but in other situations putting more stress on an arthritic joint can worsen the problem. Also in systemic or inflammatory arthritis, it is important to have regular periods of rest during the day.

♦ **10   Can I expect other organs or other joints to become involved with this type of arthritis?**

It would be nice if arthritis were limited to joints and, in some cases, it is. But in some types of arthritis, especially that which occurs in younger people, the arthritis is simply one symptom of disease caused by antibodies to one's own body parts. With time, lungs, kidneys, and other organs can be attacked, and symptoms from these areas can be expected. These may even appear before the arthritis does.

♦ **11   Should I follow a special diet?**

Diet is not usually a critical factor in arthritis, but it can be. If you are overweight, for example, stress on joints can be lessened by weight loss. Or if you have one of the systemic types of arthritis in which other organs like the kidneys are involved, diet may be important. Also, in a common type of arthritis, gout, which is caused by high levels of uric acid, diet occasionally is important.

♦ **12   Is my job as a _____ compatible with this disease, or should I consider a career change?**

Arthritis is an illness whose effects may be visible and is quite likely to have great impact on the patient's mobility and ability to do certain things. Fine finger and hand movements and picking up objects may be difficult when hands are involved; when hips, knees or ankles are affected, walking may be painful. Jobs that depend on facility with involved joints may become impossible. Early retraining or career changes should be considered. Leisure activities or hobbies that aggravate joints may also need to be curtailed.

◆ 13   Is there a chapter of The Arthritis Society in this area?

Associations devoted to helping persons with similar chronic illness can be a great help. Some of the services that such a group might provide include disseminating resource material, putting you in touch with persons with similar problems, giving you tips for maintaining joint mobility, providing information about replacement joints and information about helpful aids for persons who have disabling joint deformities.

◆ 14   Do you know of any aids to help arthritis victims do their work?

While your doctor may not himself have such devices, he should be able to refer you to someone who would have information regarding special devices to open jars, etc. Sometimes medical equipment suppliers will have this type of thing, as well as aids for getting into and out of a bathtub, wheelchairs, and special beds.

ASTHMA

◆ 1   What type of asthma do I have?

The term *asthma* refers to reversible narrowing of airways which makes breathing more difficult. A variety of causes of asthma have been identified. It will help you to understand the illness better and improve your ability to forestall acute attacks if you know what kind of asthma you have.

◆ 2   Is my asthma related to my work or exercise?

A number of materials irritate the airways and cause asthma through a variety of mechanisms. A good history of worsening of symptoms at work is needed to establish this relationship. More subtle causes like exercise or cold (e.g., a meat-packer who works in a walk-in cooler) may be the culprits.

♦ 3   **Are my children at risk for developing asthma?**

Certain types of asthma have a strong family tendency, and this is particularly true if there are allergies present. It is useful to know in advance if your children may develop asthma so that you are not caught unawares; at the same time, there is nothing specific you can do to prevent it from occurring.

♦ 4   **If my asthma is work-related, am I eligible for workers' compensation or job retraining?**

A number of factors are involved here, including strict criteria for establishing the relationship to work; however, if this relationship is shown, compensation is usually available. Compensation laws vary from one area to another, and you will have to determine what is applicable in your area.

♦ 5   **Do I need to take medications every day?**

Asthma is highly variable from one person to another, and medications are used to *prevent* acute attacks (although they also are used once an attack occurs). Many persons require medication on a daily basis for many years. Some patients who can point to specific precipitating events, like exercise or upper respiratory tract infections, can use medications only when these precipitants occur. Find out the best approach for your disease.

♦ 6   **Would some types of medication be better for me than others?**

The speed of action, the convenience of pills vs. inhalers, one's type of asthma, individual tolerances or sensitivities all may influence a decision about medication. Since a number of different types of drug are available with a number of delivery systems, discuss with your doctor which might be the best for you.

◆ **7   Do you have any suggestions for avoiding attacks?**

Obviously, avoiding precipitants is a way of avoiding attacks, but there may be other factors—specific exposures, medications for other illnesses, stress, poor compliance with medications, smoking—that are interfering with the best control.

◆ **8   Can I adjust my own medication? How?**

Many asthmatics can learn how to manipulate their medication to give the best control and keep them out of emergency rooms and reduce hospital admissions. This sort of manipulation, however, must be thoroughly discussed with the physician, since some asthma drugs can have serious toxic effects if taken in excessive doses.

◆ **9   Am I using my medications correctly? Should I be using any of the medication aids?**

Technique is very important in using many of the asthma medicines, especially the inhaled ones. Make sure you understand how to use the inhalers, and if you cannot manage this, inquire about some of the medication-administering aids available. Improper medication use is very common among asthmatics.

◆ **10   What side effects of my medications should I be watching for?**

While the usual medications for asthma, with the exception of steroids, *do not* have many serious *long-term side effects,* they may have toxic effects when used in amounts only moderately higher than recommended dosages. Clarify what toxic effects to watch for if you are getting too much of a medication. Also, make sure you understand the long-term serious side effects of steroids if you require them.

◆ **11   Should I have allergy testing or any other special tests?**

In patients whose asthma is closely related to exposure to certain substances and/or if the asthma is particularly severe, allergy testing and hyposensitization shots may be useful. This is a somewhat controversial question among physicians, but some patients seem to be particularly suited to hyposensitization therapy. Other tests may be recommended to assess and follow the asthma. These include breathing tests, chest x-rays, and sometimes arterial blood samples to assess blood oxygen levels. Also, blood tests measuring the amount of drug present may help in adjusting doses of some asthma medications.

◆ **12   Are there any particular medications I should avoid?**

This is an important question in asthma for two reasons. First, some medications for other illnesses can precipitate asthma attacks. Second, some medications can influence the amount of asthma drugs in the blood and may necessitate adjusting drug dosages.

◆ **13   Will any drugs I am taking adversely affect a pregnancy?**

Many asthmatics are young women who will have to continue drugs during pregnancy. If you fit in this category and are planning a pregnancy, make sure before you get pregnant that the drugs you are on are not known to cause birth defects.

◆ **14   What should I do if I get an asthma attack?**

Waiting until an asthma attack is well established makes it that much harder to treat and increases the chance of hospitalization. Work out clearly with your doctor what you should do early in an attack. If you have a plan in advance—whether it is to adjust medication, go to an emergency room, or call the doctor—you are likely to spend less time in a hospital, because early attacks can be aborted *and* good planning greatly reduces anxiety, a major contributor to most asthma exacerbations.

♦ 15   Do you know of any self-help groups for asthma patients?

Asthma can be very disruptive in terms of time lost from work and missed social and family occasions. Anxiety as mentioned above is often a big contributor to the illness, and in some cases, self-help groups exist for these patients. If one is available in your area, and you have had difficulty dealing with your disease, you may benefit from this. If your physician is unaware of any such groups, contact the nearest branch of the American or the Canadian Lung Association for more information.

CANCER

♦ 1   Can you draw me a diagram of this tumor and explain exactly what it is?

Visual aids often are best at clarifying one's mind and putting into perspective the cancer that has been discovered. Also, they help you understand the reason for doing the necessary studies to establish spread.

♦ 2   What sort of tests will be needed to establish whether or not the disease has spread? Do I need to be hospitalized?

Tumors nearly always have to be "staged" (have their extent determined) in order to give a prognosis and recommend the appropriate treatment. This can sometimes be done with simple tests as an outpatient. However, most often you would likely be hospitalized for a thorough evaluation and initiation of therapy.

♦ 3   How much spread of disease do the tests show and how reliable is this information?

Once testing has been done to stage the cancer, find out what the tests that were done show. Sometimes, even though negative, tests do not give a reliable indication of extent of disease. Is this so in your case? Were the tests of good quality?

♦ 4   Now that we know the size and extent of my cancer, what are my chances of cure?

Survival and "five-year disease-free" rates for all cancers are known and based on both tumor type and degree of spread at diagnosis. You can be given this type of statistic, but remember that statistics are derived from large numbers of patients and cannot be directly applied to you as a single victim.

♦ 5   Are there other currently accepted alternative approaches to the therapy of this cancer?

Your doctor will probably recommend the therapy he uses for a specific type of cancer. There may be other approaches being used by reputable doctors that are equally effective but more acceptable to you. This might be, for example, a chemotherapy protocol causing temporary hair loss vs. one that does not. In breast cancer, it might involve a "lumpectomy" vs. a modified radical mastectomy.

♦ 6   Are any family members at risk for this kind of cancer?

Some tumors seem to be more common in certain families, and some familial diseases (like polyposis of the colon) predispose to cancers. This information is important for monitoring of persons at risk, since tumors picked up early are, of course, more easily treated.

♦ 7   Is this cancer related to any drug, smoke, chemical, or other environmental exposure?

Certain drugs and chemicals are known to increase one's chance of cancer, and smoking greatly increases one's risk of lung cancer. You may want to know this both for reasons of compensation, as well as pointing out the danger to others in hazardous situations.

The following sets of questions relate directly to the major types of therapy given and will be relevant only if you are undergoing that type of treatment.

CHEMOTHERAPY

♦ 1   What drug(s) will I be receiving and how are they given?

The effective drugs vary from cancer to cancer and what is used varies from hospital to hospital, depending on what regimens are currently employed, unless one drug (or a group of drugs) has clearly been shown to be superior to others. That two people with the same illness get different drugs does not mean one protocol is better than the other. The drugs may be taken by mouth or given intravenously, or occasionally by other methods. The more you know before your therapy, the less anxiety you will feel when you are treated.

♦ 2   What are the chances the drugs will be effective in my cancer?

Published reports will generally be available stating the percentage of tumors similar to yours that have responded to this therapy. Ask whether a response is likely to mean complete obliteration of the tumor or not, and how long the response is likely to last if only partial obliteration is achieved. You can get a reasonable idea about whether or not the drugs are expected to be "curative," which generally means apparent complete eradication of the tumor for at least five years.

♦ 3   How do you measure the effectiveness of treatment?

Whether or not a treatment is working can be assessed in several ways. Symptoms may improve, tumor masses may shrink, blood or other tests may change. Be prepared to undergo repeated tests (often several times) to measure effect of therapy. Discuss with your physician which tests will be necessary, and you won't be surprised by what needs to be done during the course of the therapy.

♦ **4   Will I have any side effects from the drugs as soon as I get therapy or within a few days or weeks?**

Cancer drugs are notoriously toxic, though some may have little or no immediate discomfort associated. Nausea and vomiting are the most often seen immediate effects, and these can usually be controlled. Other effects, e.g., mouth ulcers and hair loss, occur days to weeks later. If you know what may occur, you will be better prepared to handle it if it does.

♦ **5   Can I receive my chemotherapy as an outpatient or must I be hospitalized?**

Many cancers can be treated with outpatient therapy if they do not require long intravenous infusions and if the patient has tolerated initial doses well. If it is your wish to be treated as an outpatient, make that known, and your doctor will probably make every effort to accommodate you.

♦ **6   Will other organs be damaged by the chemotherapy, and if so, what long-term effects might occur?**

Chemotherapeutic drugs do not specifically kill tumor cells; they simply kill more tumor cells than normal body cells. Most body cells do not replicate often enough to be damaged by the drugs. Nevertheless, many long-term toxic effects can result from chemotherapy. These may vary from drug to drug, but can include, among other things, heart damage, sterility, lung disease, development of other types of cancer.

♦ **7   Will I be prone to infections, and if so, what symptoms should I watch for?**

Some drugs much more than others depress the bone marrow, which contains red and white blood cells, and predispose to life-threatening infections. If your chemotherapy includes these types of drug, find out what symptoms should alert you—e.g., any fever, muscle aches, shortness of breath—to a serious infection and to the need of emergency evaluation.

♦ 8   **Should I limit my work or life-style during chemotherapy?**

Aside from general feelings of fatigue, your doctors may wish for you to take long periods of rest and limit activities during chemotherapy, or they may not. Clarify this before you begin treatment.

RADIATION THERAPY

♦ 1   **Please explain to me what will take place during the radiation.**

To know in advance where and how the radiation is done will allay your anxiety considerably.

♦ 2   **What body areas will be radiated?**

Sometimes only the area where a tumor mass is located is radiated, but other areas may be radiated to prevent emergence of tumor there, e.g., the brain. Ask about this so that you are not caught unaware. Discuss this with your doctor in advance, since you may have temporary hair loss or other side effects.

♦ 3   **How many doses of radiation will I receive and over what period of time?**

Radiation is given in different ways for different tumors, for different intended results or in different medical centers. You may not get exactly the same therapy as someone somewhere else with the same tumor; if this is the case, it is because neither treatment has been shown to be superior to the other.

♦ 4   **Is this therapy considered palliative or curative?**

Radiation often is given to improve symptoms though it is known to be not curative in a particular situation; other times it is given, usually in larger doses, as a curative therapy. Clarify your situation so you have no misunderstandings about the outcome.

♦ 5   **What are the immediate and long-term side effects related to radiation in the areas that will be covered?**

As with chemotherapy, immediate and long-term effects can vary from uncomfortable to life-threatening. Whereas in chemotherapy risks often vary most from drug to drug and increase with higher doses, in radiation therapy risks are related most to areas involved directly by the radiation and the doses used. Again, side effects like organ damage and sterility can be seen.

SURGERY

♦ 1   Is this surgery aimed at cure? If not, will it help extend or improve my life?

Surgery where possible is most often used as a curative effort. Occasionally, it is used to prevent a life-threatening complication and is not expected to produce a cure. Other times, once the surgery is under way and the tumor is visualized, it becomes obvious it cannot be completely removed and a palliative procedure is done.

♦ 2   Can you draw a diagram to help me understand where the tumor is and what you expect to do?

Whether it is lung, bowel, uterus, stomach, or whatever, it often helps you to prepare for surgery if you understand what the surgeon expects to do. The prospect of surgery is very frightening, and decreasing your fears in any way you can is important.

♦ 3   Will I have any deformities or disabilities as a result of surgery?

Surgery for cancer can result in loss of breast, loss of limb, formation of an opening for the bowel in the abdominal wall (colostomy), and other things. Avoid being surprised when you wake because you didn't ask enough questions before surgery.

♦ 4   What is the risk of death or serious complications with surgery?

Depending on underlying diseases, age, and other factors, the risk of serious postoperative problems or death may be high. Chances of cure may not be high enough to justify the risks.

♦ 5   **What is the usual recovery time from this type of surgery?**

Knowing expected recovery time back to "normal" life will help you plan better and avoid unrealistic expectations.

MULTIPLE THERAPIES / NO THERAPY

♦ 1   **Would I benefit from multiple types of therapy?**

Often nowadays, cancers are treated with at least two and sometimes more types of therapy, sometimes at the same time and sometimes sequentially. This varies both with extent and type of tumor, i.e., whether your cancer is one that requires multiple modality therapy.

♦ 2   **Will the chemotherapeutic drugs pose any additional problems with radiation?**

Often combined therapies are indicated for cancers. Sometimes, drugs used increase the potency of radiation, or vice versa, and the toxic effects can be magnified also.

♦ 3   **If I elect to choose no therapy, what is my likely survival? What is it with therapy?**

No one will be able to answer exactly, but if you have heard of the relative success rates vs. the complications of therapy and are unimpressed, you always have the option of no therapy. Be sure you have a full understanding of the alternatives, however, before you choose this course.

♦ 4   **Should I have a particular diet or nutritional supplements?**

Wasting is one of the most insidious, constant and difficult to attack accompaniments of cancer. However, knowing what to eat and how to add as many calories as possible can be helpful in stemming weight loss. Ask your doctor for a visit to a dietitian or nutritionist.

◆ 5 How active should I be?

Once you feel able after therapy, most doctors feel you should resume as active a life as possible. Ask if you have any particular circumstances in which this is inadvisable.

BEYOND TREATMENT

◆ 1 If the disease progresses despite therapy, what type of problems or disabilities can I expect?

Different cancers as they grow have different patterns of spread and cause different complications. The doctor can probably tell you some general problems you may encounter and how to deal with them, but he cannot predict exactly what will happen in your specific case.

◆ 2 If I develop suddenly painful or otherwise distressing complications, what should I do?

As your disease progresses, discuss the types of care you wish at what stages of the disease, and who you contact in case of emergency. If or when an emergency arises, you should discuss potential palliative measures fully to decide to what lengths you wish to go to prolong your life and what the likely quality of your life will be in the various circumstances.

◆ 3 Are there any support groups in my area for patients/families with this cancer?

Support groups can be of tremendous help in dealing with the psychosocial impact of cancer, as well as the day-to-day insults of the disease. Several have been formed and probably have chapters in your area.

◆ 4 If my care becomes very difficult for myself or my family, are there any hospitals or other facilities for which I would be eligible, and how do I apply?

Many areas have facilities particularly for cancer patients. The end stages of the disease may pose care problems and tensions that you never thought possible in the family. It is wise to be aware of and apply for this type of facility if it may be necessary.

◆ **5   If I become terminally ill, will you honor my request for (a) no artificial life support, (b) full life support?**

Find out the philosophy of your physician early and make sure it is agreeable to you. If you wish no artificial life support but the physician does not feel comfortable with this view, this may become a big source of dissension. Find someone who is more in agreement with your wishes for your treatment as death approaches. Likewise, if you want every possible thing done and your physician is not agreeable, this could also cause major problems.

◆ **6   If I develop severe pain, can I be assured of receiving whatever medication is necessary to control it?**

While pain is not an inevitable complication of cancer, it can be. If pain is a likely component of your illness, find out how your doctor deals with this type of problem if it becomes severe and unrelenting. Knowing his approach and that he will alleviate pain will give you some peace of mind regarding one of the fears most often mentioned by cancer victims.

CORONARY ARTERY DISEASE

◆ **1   Can you draw a picture showing me where the blood vessels to my heart are narrowed or closed?**

If you have had a heart catheterization done, the doctor should be able to draw an accurate picture for you; a diagram will give you something concrete to understand. Even if your diagnosis has been based on other studies or symptoms, the doctor can make a general illustration of the problem.

♦ **2   Have I had permanent damage to my heart, and if so, what does it mean to me?**

You may or may not have had a heart attack (myocardial infarction), in which some heart muscle has died, and a scar has formed. Even without a heart attack, you may have evidence through other studies that tissue damage is present. This may have importance regarding activities, medications, future problems.

♦ **3   What post–heart attack complications might I develop?**

Depending upon the size of the damaged muscle, region of heart involved, and individual factors, you may be at risk for developing complications in the days, weeks, or months after the heart attack. If you know in advance what might happen, you will know what symptoms to be watching for.

♦ **4   How do I recognize these complications and when should I contact you?**

For your peace of mind, establish a plan for communication and follow-up after your heart attack. Learn the symptoms of problems that might develop. These might include, for example, chest pain, swelling of ankles, shortness of breath, or palpitations. Your particular situation should be discussed with the doctor.

♦ **5   Should I have a cardiac catheterization or coronary artery bypass surgery (heart vessel surgery)?**

A variety of factors which vary from patient to patient enter into this decision. The fact that your neighbor has had heart surgery for his coronary artery disease but it is not recommended for you may mean that his heart disease is quite different from yours, e.g., his heart attack occurred in a different area and therefore involved different vessels, he has ongoing pain, he has problems with rhythm.

♦ **6   Should I be taking heart medications and, if so, what for?**

Different types of medications may be given for a variety of reasons—rhythm disturbances, heart failure, pain—to try to prevent further heart damage. Clarify what each medication you have is supposed to do and exactly how to take it.

◆ 7   What are the expected results from these medicines? Should I be looking for specific end points, and how should these be evaluated?

Medicines may be expected to totally control symptoms, but often that is unrealistic and some lesser goal is set, say 80 percent of rhythm disturbances or pain episodes. Some end points may be monitored by repeated tests, others by your assessment of symptoms. Generally, heart medicines control symptoms, they do not cure. However, some drugs may be given in the hope they will reduce risk of heart attack.

◆ 8   What are the side effects of the medication I am taking, and what symptoms should I report to you?

Most heart medicines have some minor side effects and occasionally more severe ones. With some, a toxic level of drug is not much greater than the recommended doses. Understand what side effects you should expect and which require modification of therapy.

◆ 9   Do these medicines interact with other medicines I am taking or other diseases I have?

Heart disease can be a complication of other illness (e.g., diabetes) or coexist with other illness (e.g., chronic obstructive lung disease), and the medications used for controlling symptoms may have an undesirable impact on the other illness or with other medicines used. This does not necessarily mean such drugs should not be used; it merely means monitoring or at least awareness of potential problems may have to increase. For example, propranolol or similar drugs are often used in the treatment of coronary artery disease and these same drugs can worsen asthma. If both diseases are present in the same person, propranolol may have to be used carefully or not at all.

♦ **10   How long should I expect to take medication?**

Some cardiac medications are meant to be taken only for short periods; others for life. Find out why your medicines are prescribed for you and if reaching the end point of therapy means you can discontinue the drug.

♦ **11   If you are recommending heart surgery, why and what type of results can I expect? What is the success rate?**

Surgery may be a coronary artery bypass graft (CABG) aimed at pain relief or it may be one of several types of surgery designed to get rid of rhythm disturbances or other problems. A separate problem may be diseased heart valves that are to be replaced. Whatever the reason, make sure you understand clearly the aims of surgery and the chance of success so you can make a reasonable decision about going ahead with it.

♦ **12   What are the risks to me of this surgery?**

The risks of the surgery, aside from the anesthesia and surgery itself, depend to some degree on your age, the extent of your disease and underlying illnesses, especially chest disease. Make sure the surgical risks are clear.

♦ **13   What is my risk of another heart attack with or without surgery?**

Statistics can now predict whether or not surgery has any impact on the occurrence of future myocardial infarctions and mortality. The location of the diseased blood vessels, the extent of the diseased vessels, and individual risk factors are important. However, do not expect the doctor to predict what will happen in your specific situation. He can only give statistics.

♦ **14   Are there any diet or life-style changes that will reduce my chances of developing or worsening my heart disease?**

You may already be on an appropriate diet, do not smoke, and have reduced the high-stress events in your life. On the other hand, you may have a variety of nutritional and daily habits that are aggravating your heart condition. Preventive medicine is something you can do for yourself and it's the best approach.

◆ **15 Do you know of a rehabilitation program or exercise class for persons with my type of heart disease?**

Many cardiac rehabilitation programs exist for patients who suffer from coronary artery disease or have undergone open heart surgery. If your doctor does not know of any, the local hospital or local chapter of the American Heart Association or Canadian Heart Foundation will.

◆ **16 Will I be able to have sexual intercourse without risking another heart attack?**

The answer to this is usually yes, although you should clarify your particular circumstances with your physician. Often some modification of your usual sexual relations can be made if you cannot tolerate the usual activity levels.

◆ **17 Will I be able to return to my job as a _____, and how soon?**

Most patients often return to work relatively soon after a heart attack, an episode of prolonged chest pain, or heart surgery. Your particular job, however, if stressful, may make your return more difficult. This should be discussed in detail with your doctor.

◆ **18 Are relaxation techniques useful?**

It is easy to become overly anxious, once one has had a heart attack, that another is going to occur and to become basically housebound. Learning to relax a bit can help patients with this problem. There may be someone in your area who does this type of teaching; some educational material is probably available as well from your local chapter of the American Heart Association or the Canadian Heart Foundation.

◆ **19 Do I have any risk factors that are genetic or environmental, and can my family members do anything to reduce their risk of heart attacks?**

A number of risk factors are genetic, but continuous treatment from an early age will decrease, though not eliminate, the chance of heart disease in family members at risk. Smoking, stress, and a variety of other environmental hazards can significantly increase one's chance of heart disease. Most of these environmental hazards can be avoided.

DIABETES MELLITUS

♦ 1   **Please explain what type of diabetes I have.**

Diabetes mellitus refers to an illness in which the blood sugar is abnormally high, but several different causes and types of diabetes exist. These may have quite divergent prognoses with respect to complications, heredity, treatment, and other factors. Occasionally, for example, diabetes may be precipitated by drugs or pregnancy, and will resolve when these factors are no longer present. Rather than a *primary* illness, diabetes may be secondary to some other disease. Even within the primary type of diabetes, several different subtypes are identified.

♦ 2   **Will I need insulin or an oral drug for blood sugar control?**

Depending on the type of diabetes, the patient's age, whether he or she is overweight, the level of the blood sugar, and a number of other factors, a special diet may be the only initial attempt at control. Insulin or a drug taken by mouth may be used. In any case, you can get an idea of what the physician feels will ultimately be needed to control your blood sugar.

♦ 3   **Will I need to be hospitalized to start my diabetic therapy?**

A patient who needs diet or oral drugs only usually does not require hospitalization for initial therapy. However, if insulin is necessary, it may be advisable to be hospitalized until the appropriate dose is achieved, since it is possible to overshoot and create a state of low blood sugar.

♦ 4   What type of glucose monitoring should I use and what guidelines should I follow?

Glucose (sugar) can be monitored either in the blood or in the urine. Most diabetics can test the urine and get adequate readings, though these are not as precise as blood sugar monitoring. A new easy method of testing blood sugar levels has been developed, and most patients can be trained to do this. It is an accurate test of the blood for glucose levels, and some diabetics may require this type of home monitoring to be able to follow their blood sugar precisely enough. Evidence is accumulating that close control of blood sugar level may help prevent some diabetic complications. Be sure you understand completely how monitoring is done and what guidelines you should follow.

♦ 5   Please explain the diabetic diet to me.

Many diabetics can achieve adequate control of their blood sugar level by adhering to a strict diet. However, often because of misunderstanding, the diabetic patient does not follow the diet. If you are at all unsure about instructions, ask for a repeat explanation. A thorough understanding from the beginning can prevent hospitalizations later.

♦ 6   When my home monitoring reveals values outside the guidelines, what should I do?

It is critical to know what to do with the results of home monitoring. Establish whether or not you can adjust your own medication, and under what circumstances you should contact your doctor.

♦ 7   Will the drugs I am taking for other illnesses interfere with my diabetes in any way?

Other drugs or illnesses may cause blood sugars to become high or low, or prevent the usual symptoms one gets from low blood sugar. To be informed about your health, you must understand potential interactions of medications and illnesses. Occasionally, these can be overlooked by your doctor unless you specifically mention them.

♦ 8   What are the chances of developing complications, and what are they?

While it is impossible to predict who will develop the often disabling complications of diabetes (including blindness, kidney failure, nerve abnormalities, heart disease, and others), in certain situations complications may develop more often than in others. In addition, less commonly recognized but very disturbing complications like diarrhea and impotence are possible. Your doctor should evaluate the risks and discuss whether he feels close control of your blood sugar level will help.

♦ 9   If I develop complications, what are the chances of these occurring during my active work life?

It often takes a number of years for complications to develop, and the complications may be more likely in certain types of diabetes. This is critical to know, since some complications may impair your ability to work in certain occupations.

♦ 10   If complications occur, are they likely to affect my ability to work as a _____ ?

It may seem that a lot of questions are directed toward complications, but in fact the complications of diabetes can be devastating to your ability to do your job. You should be completely informed about possible complications early in your disease, so decisions can be made about retraining or redirecting your career if that is appropriate.

♦ 11   Can I prevent complications from occurring?

Much diabetes research is directed toward preventing complications. Keep up to date with your doctor about any new information that suggests ways to prevent complications. Currently, the thought is that maintaining near-normal values of blood sugar may decrease some types of complications, but this is still an area of much research.

♦ 12   Should I be considered for any of the new blood sugar control measures like insulin pumps or special insulins?

A few patients with special problems may benefit from experimental or "new" therapeutic techniques. Sometimes these are used for patients with hard-to-control blood sugars, pregnant women, unusually early or difficult complications, etc. You may have a problem that fits into one of these categories.

♦ 13   What therapy is available to treat my complications?

This question is really not pertinent unless you already have advanced disease, since the modes of therapy are changing all the time. Some therapies—ranging from laser treatment for some eye complications to kidney transplant for kidney failure, and penile implants for impotence—are currently available but are mostly palliative.

♦ 14   On a day-to-day basis, what can cause dangerously high or low blood sugars? What should I do if one of these circumstances occurs?

It is important to know causes of high and low blood sugars because either can result in physical damage or death. This might include forgetting your insulin, a severe episode of flu or a cold, etc. Make sure you know and understand in your case the most likely causes, so you can try to avoid those circumstances. Also, have a plan to follow for increased monitoring, etc., that you have discussed with the doctor in case of any of these circumstances.

♦ 15   What are the symptoms of dangerously high or low sugars, and what should I do when I feel I am experiencing them?

Diabetes is an illness that requires constant vigilance. You should be aware of symptoms to watch for and get detailed instructions about what to do if you should experience them.

♦ **16   Will the fact I have diabetes affect my health and/or life insurance or insurability?**

Because of the possible long-term problems associated with diabetes, insurability may be a problem. Premiums may be increased in certain circumstances. You may wish to contact your local diabetes association or your doctor for guidance if you run into problems with your insurability.

♦ **17   What problems do I and my child face if I become pregnant?**

Pregnancy in diabetic women has become increasingly safe when the women have close monitoring and blood sugars are kept near normal, but they must be very closely followed. Be sure to find out early what steps must be followed to ensure a safe pregnancy.

♦ **18   Is there a chapter of the American or Canadian Diabetes Association nearby?**

This "illness" association is one of the most active and has many services from which diabetics can benefit, as well as many ways in which you can contribute to furthering the understanding and research into this illness.

EMPHYSEMA / CHRONIC BRONCHITIS

♦ **1   Please explain the cause of my lung disease.**

The cause of most emphysema and chronic bronchitis is smoking, though a small percentage of patients may have disease of unknown cause, hereditary disease, or disease resulting from other known factors.

♦ **2   Will changing my environment or life-style factors improve my illness?**

Smoking obviously worsens these chronic lung illnesses, but other factors might also be important, e.g., living in a city with high pollution levels, working in jobs in which much dust is in the air. Sometimes, changing environmental factors will improve or at least stop the progression of symptoms.

♦ 3   Is my disease hereditary?

Some types of emphysema are hereditary and can be tested for in susceptible patients. Smoking worsens the disease in these patients, so it is valuable to know this early and try to reduce the rate of progression of disease.

♦ 4   Would I benefit from medications?

Though these illnesses are often considered irreversible, sometimes medications do considerably improve the patient's ability to breathe. Often, even when breathing tests before and after medication show no obvious improvement, doctors will try medication anyway because often patients seem to experience some relief of symptoms. Usually used are drugs called bronchodilators, which open up the tubelike airways, the bronchi.

♦ 5   Should I worry about interactions of the medications with drugs I am taking for another disease?

Medications for other illnesses may influence the amount of some drugs in the blood and the length of time these drugs stay in the blood. This can be a problem with some medications for lung disease in which the difference between therapeutic and toxic levels is not great. Other interactions may also be present.

♦ 6   Should I receive influenza or antipneumonia vaccinations?

Since these illnesses can be fatal in patients with significant lung disease, most doctors immunize such patients. On the other hand, you may have some specific reason why you should not receive such a vaccination, e.g., an allergy to it.

♦ **7 Aside from medications, are there any exercises or other steps I can take to improve my functioning?**

Breathing exercises, graded exercise, nutritional and other education are all a part of an increasing number of respiratory rehabilitation programs.

♦ **8 Is there an organized rehabilitation program in my area?**

There are a growing number of these efforts sponsored by local hospitals, lung associations, and veterans' hospitals. Both outpatient and inpatient programs are available. To find out if your area has one, ask your doctor or contact the local chapter of the American or Canadian Lung Association.

♦ **9 Should I be tested for supplemental oxygen?**

Certain standards are generally adhered to for the prescribing of this expensive drug. If you have a significant amount of lung impairment, you may need oxygen at least part of the day. You will probably need to undergo a series of evaluations to determine how much and for how many hours per day. Mild disease does not require oxygen. Oxygen is not given simply for breathlessness, which may not reflect the level of oxygen in the blood.

♦ **10 Am I at risk traveling to high altitude or in an airplane?**

Patients who have significantly lowered blood oxygen levels may feel worse when traveling to higher altitudes or in airplanes which are not pressurized to sea level. If you intend to travel, be sure to tell your doctor and arrange for oxygen supplies if necessary.

♦ **11 What should I do if I get a cold or any changes in my breathing?**

Get clear instructions from your doctor about what specific symptoms to be alarmed about, what you can do to handle the situation yourself and for how long, and when you should report to an emergency room. This is particularly important for patients with severe lung disease who have little lung reserve and can become deathly ill very quickly.

♦ **12   If I require surgery for some reason, am I at increased risk because of my lung disease?**

The severity of some complicating illnesses, such as pneumonia, is often increased when a person already has damaged lungs.

Lung disease, especially when severe, poses a much increased risk in surgery. Less severe disease may not increase the risk at all. This should be discussed early with your doctor in case an emergency situation arises. Preplanning can assure that in a surgical setting, the best preparations and decisions can be made to ensure postoperative survival.

♦ **13   Should I have periodic evaluation of my lung function and blood oxygen level?**

While periodic tests may not *help* your disease, they are of little risk and do give useful information about the progression of your illness. They are also useful as a baseline to compare with values when you become acutely ill or if your risks for surgery are being evaluated.

♦ **14   Is there a chapter of the American (or Canadian) Lung Association in this area?**

Self-help groups, educational information, and other services are available through this organization. The concentration of energy in the lung association is on the diseases caused by smoking, since they are the most common lung diseases.

HEPATITIS AND/OR CIRRHOSIS OF THE LIVER

♦ **1   What is the cause of my liver disease?**

Hepatitis/cirrhosis has a large number of causes that can include, among others, drugs, alcohol, viruses, and genetic factors. Your doctor will make every effort to learn the cause to prevent possible transmission of the disease as well as to try to limit the damage.

◆ 2   **How can I avoid passing this illness to others?**

Infectious hepatitis is spread by body fluids (hepatitis B) or fecal-oral means (hepatitis A). Certain measures need to be taken by infected persons to prevent transmission of illness. Other forms of hepatitis are generally not transmissible. If the illness is infectious, ask how long you are likely to remain contagious and what the incubation period is, so that you know how long to take precautions and watch for symptoms in close personal contacts. A more recently discovered infectious hepatitis called non-A, non-B seems to be spread by blood products, mostly through transfusions.

◆ 3   **If not infectious, what is the most likely cause of this disease?**

Many drugs have effects on the liver. The most common of these is alcohol, but the range of offenders includes many prescription drugs. Make sure the doctor is aware of all medications you take, even on an occasional basis. Other causes include complications of your other medical problems, tumors and so on.

◆ 4   **Will a liver biopsy or other procedure be needed to definitely establish a diagnosis?**

Blood tests done after you report symptoms of hepatitis will confirm the illness, but occasionally a liver biopsy or other tests need to be done to confirm the precise cause and to assess the extent of damage. You should know if this is recommended, as it will probably require a short hospitalization and may entail some risk.

◆ 5   **What is the prognosis of my type of hepatitis, and can I do anything to alter that prognosis?**

The cause of the hepatitis makes a great difference in whether it may go on to cirrhosis, or scarring of the liver.

In many cases if the cause, e.g., alcohol, can be found and eliminated, the prognosis can be changed for the better.

◆ 6   **Is there any treatment for my liver disease?**

Some chronic forms of hepatitis or cirrhosis are treated with some success with drugs like steroids or drugs that suppress the immune system. You may be a candidate for this kind of therapy. Other drugs aimed at improving symptoms may be used in cirrhosis. However, once cirrhosis is established, the scarring that diagnosis implies cannot be reversed.

◆ 7   **If I have drug-related liver disease, does that mean I must never take that drug again?**

Sometimes a drug causes liver problems because of other concurrent problems. Sometimes it is toxic only because it is used in combination with other drugs, or sometimes because of the dose used. This may be an important drug for you, and if any of the preceding situations apply, you may be able to take this drug in the future if circumstances change.

◆ 8   **Will my hepatitis/cirrhosis necessitate changing the doses of other medications I take?**

Anything that interferes with liver function may increase blood levels of other medications to toxic levels, because many drugs are cleared from the body by the liver. Discuss this with your doctor so appropriate dose adjustments can be made.

◆ 9   **Will I likely have relapses, and how will I know it?**

Some forms of hepatitis have relapsing courses. When a relapse occurs, certain symptoms may appear and some precautions (e.g., adjustment of medications) may need to be undertaken. Be aware of the warning signs.

◆ 10   **Regardless of the cause of my liver disease, should I avoid alcohol?**

Some doctors feel that regardless of the cause of hepatitis, alcohol is a liver toxin and should be avoided if there is any evidence of liver disease.

♦ **11   Am I at risk for developing chronic disease or cirrhosis?**

While this type of question can never be answered with complete certainty, some types of hepatitis are known to be more likely to progress to cirrhosis. Certainly continued use of a damaging drug will lead to further liver damage. A biopsy or other tests can be used to give a reasonable answer.

♦ **12   Should I be on a special diet?**

Patients with cirrhosis may be able to avoid or minimize some complications of their disease by adhering to special diets. Dietitians in your local hospital will be able to outline an appropriate diet if it is indicated.

♦ **13   Am I at risk for developing other complications? What are they?**

Patients with hepatitis or cirrhosis can have many difficulties, depending on the severity of their disease, infections that may arise, dietary indiscretions, etc. Be aware of symptoms to look for and, if possible, measures to take to avoid complications.

♦ **14   Will I be able to work at my job as a _____?**

Complete recovery from hepatitis of the various types usually does not impair one's employability. Chronic hepatitis or cirrhosis often leaves you easily fatigued, and strenuous jobs may be difficult to maintain. Persons with hepatitis type B, in some cases, continue to be carriers of the disease and can pass the disease to others through body fluid or blood. However, in very few occupations would this be of serious concern.

♦ **15   If I have a progressive disease, would I be a candidate for a liver transplant?**

Liver transplantation is now a real possibility for some patients suffering terminal liver disease. However, many restrictions still apply to patients who are selected, and a transplant brings other types of complications, as well as a lifelong need for immune suppression medication to prevent the body from rejecting the liver. It's much better to avoid reaching this point if at all possible.

HIGH BLOOD PRESSURE
(Hypertension)

♦ 1   What is the cause of my high blood pressure?

While most cases of high blood pressure are considered "essential" (without any specific cause), a few identifiable and correctable causes are known. Usually, there are tipoffs to these: unusual symptoms, age of onset, abnormal blood values, etc.

♦ 2   Should an intravenous pyelogram (IVP) or other investigations be done to further look for causes of my hypertension?

Often the work-up for high blood pressure is quite minimal if it is felt to be "essential." However, if you have characteristics that are unusual in patients with essential hypertension, you may need an evaluation to search for specific correctable causes. Specific kidney problems are the most common, so often the first study done is an x-ray dye study of the kidney called an intravenous pyelogram.

♦ 3   Is the high blood pressure related to my other medical problems or medications, and does this change the prognosis?

High blood pressure can develop as a side effect of drug therapy or as a complication of other chronic illnesses. Often when it develops as a complication of other illness, it reflects involvement of the kidney by that illness, and this may mean a worse prognosis.

♦ 4   Can I make life-style or diet changes that will allow me to control my high blood pressure without medication?

Mild essential hypertension in obese persons can sometimes be controlled by weight loss and maintenance of a low-salt diet; in others, following a low-salt diet may be adequate. The patient who follows this approach has to adhere closely to the diet, though, and must maintain the weight loss, as the hypertension is a lifelong problem once it is detected. If you are going to try to control high blood pressure this way, you should be monitored often to make sure it is successful.

♦ 5 **Please explain how the medication you are prescribing works.**

Most times, therapy is started with a diuretic (water pill), but if this is inadequate, a variety of other medications with a variety of other mechanisms are available. When multiple medications are used, usually they work by different mechanisms.

♦ 6 **Should I have potassium supplementation?**

Water pills (diuretics) will cause a loss of potassium from the body as the salt is lost in the urine. Depending on the patient and the type and amount of diuretic used, as well as the patient's diet, potassium supplements may or may not be needed. Periodic blood tests may be required to assess this.

♦ 7 **Will the drugs I am taking for hypertension interact with my other medications or influence my other medical problems?**

This is often an issue in the treatment of high blood pressure. Because hypertension is such a common disease, it is often seen in patients with other medical problems, and some of the antihypertensive drugs can have important effects on other diseases. Certain antihypertensive drugs, for example, can mask low blood sugar symptoms in diabetics, precipitate asthma attacks, and worsen peptic ulcers; other drugs are available that do not produce these effects. It is critical for your doctor to know about all your medical problems and drugs so that inadvertent errors in prescribed medications do not occur.

♦ **8** **Are there any long-term side effects that may develop?**

Remember that high blood pressure, once established, is a lifelong disease and requires lifelong therapy to prevent its devastating complications, particularly heart disease, strokes, and kidney damage. Thus, you will be embarking on years of therapy with the drugs you are taking. Find out if any serious long-term side effects or toxicities from the drugs are known and how long the drugs have been used. New drugs often have not been around long enough to know all the long-term effects; be sure to keep asking your doctor if reports of any new serious side effects have been published.

♦ **9** **Can any of the drugs I am on cause impotence?**

Impotence is a big problem in the therapy of high blood pressure in that the same mechanisms that reduce pressure in blood vessels can also impair erections. The drugs that do this, however, may cause the problem in only a fraction of the patients that take the medication. Alternate medications are usually available if impotence occurs, and you can be switched to one of these. The worst thing to do, however, is to just stop taking medication if impotence occurs, because the blood pressure will quickly assume its previous, premedication level. And the patients taking these types of drugs often have blood pressures that are dangerously elevated without medication.

♦ **10** **How often should I have follow-up blood pressure checks?**

This often varies markedly from patient to patient. Patients with mild or easily controlled hypertension can be seen every several months. Others with marked hypertension, fluctuating readings, or medication problems may need weekly or biweekly follow-up and medication adjustment. Your needs may be quite different from others you know who also are being treated for high blood pressure.

♦ **11** **What if I miss some drug doses?**

Forgetting to take your medications is bound to happen once in a while. Find out if there is any danger from missing pills, like "rebound" high blood pressure. Also find out what you should do if you miss one or two doses of a drug. If you are on a two or three times a day dosing schedule, ask if there is a medication you could take once a day if you have difficulty remembering to take pills.

♦ 12   Am I in any danger if I take an extra dose by mistake?

Occasionally you may forget whether or not you have had your medication and take it again. In most instances, this is harmless, but with some medications an extra dose could conceivably drop your blood pressure excessively. If you take drugs like this, make sure you know it so you can be particularly careful.

♦ 13   Will my children be prone to high blood pressure?

The tendency to have high blood pressure can be familial. If your children are at risk, they can develop the disease while young adults and should have periodic blood pressure measurements.

♦ 14   Does my high blood pressure or the medication I am on cause risks to me or my child if I get pregnant?

High blood pressure can be a serious risk during pregnancy. While the effects of some antihypertensive drugs on fetuses are not known, make sure the drugs you are taking have not been specifically associated with birth defects. If you require medication and wish to get pregnant, you may be able to switch to a safer drug.

KIDNEY DISEASE

♦ 1   What is the underlying cause of my kidney disease?

No matter what the illness or its severity, the key to understanding its physical impact is to understand the basic disturbance. Kidney failure may result from many diverse illnesses that involve other organs of the body, or it may be the result of one of many illnesses directly attacking the kidneys.

◆ **2   Can this illness be passed on to children?**

Some types of kidney disease are hereditary. If this is a type of disease that results in total kidney failure, you may wish to have genetic counseling to predict risk in offspring.

◆ **3   Is this kidney disease part of a more generalized illness or a complication of another illness?**

The kidney, of all organs, seems to be often a target of complications or often involved as part of a generalized illness. If this role is recognized early, drug therapy directed at the basic illness may lessen risk of complications. You should be aware of the possibility of kidney involvement if you have certain illnesses, as well as the prognosis when the kidney is involved.

◆ **4   Would other special studies, such as a kidney biopsy, be of help in diagnosis or therapy? If a biopsy is advisable, am I at a particular risk?**

Biopsy or other less invasive tests may be very important in establishing a diagnosis and guiding therapy; other times they are of little use. If a biopsy is proposed, be sure you understand the potential benefits and risks, and balance the two.

◆ **5   Is my kidney disease likely to progress, and if so, how fast?**

In some illnesses, it is known approximately how fast kidney disease progresses once it is present. In others, possibility of or rate of progression is quite variable. Sometimes certain factors can be pointed to as "good" or "bad" as far as prognosis and rate of progression.

◆ **6   Should I be on a special diet or on certain drugs to help slow or reverse kidney destruction?**

Recent evidence suggests certain diets may help slow the progression of kidney disease. If your disease is part of a more generalized illness, drugs may be important in controlling the illness.

♦ **7 Should I avoid any drugs or change dosage?**

Many drugs have ill effects on the kidneys. Find out which you should avoid. Also, dosages may have to be modified because an impaired kidney will not remove drugs from the blood as well. This is a very important point for you to clarify with respect to any drugs you are taking.

♦ **8 What are the side effects of any drugs I have to take for my kidney disease?**

Drugs for diseases that cause kidney failure are often quite toxic. Find out the side effects before you begin therapy and any ways to modify potential side effects.

♦ **9 What signs or symptoms should I be watching for that might suggest worsening kidney function?**

Patients with kidney disease may live with their illness for many years, as it may worsen very slowly. If you are in this group, you should be aware of the sorts of problems or symptoms that will alert you to deteriorating kidney function and the impending need for dialysis or other therapy. Also, be aware of particular situations that might worsen previously stable or slowly progressive kidney disease. It is a good idea to contact your local chapter of the Kidney Foundation for support and for information about your illness and how to prepare for the future.

♦ **10 Will I be facing kidney dialysis?**

If your kidney function is continuing to deteriorate despite attempts to stem the loss of function, your doctor may be able to give you an idea of when you will need dialysis.

♦ **11 If I am facing dialysis, can we discuss the different types and which would be best for my disease and life-style?**

Before you get to the point of actually needing dialysis, discuss with your doctor the various types now available and think about—once you know the pros and cons—which you could handle the best or would prefer. The dialysis technique is more likely to be successful if you take an active role.

♦ **12 Would I be a candidate for a kidney transplant? When?**

Dialysis is often best as a temporary measure in kidney failure, since kidney transplants are now very successful. However, certain factors unique to you make you a good or poor candidate for transplant. Also, explore the possibilities of a relative donating a kidney to you. If there is a good tissue match, transplants from relatives are the most successful.

♦ **13 What are the problems related to transplantation in my case?**

Transplants are far from a simple cure and patients require long-term immune suppression with potential future complications, including risk of unusual infections and tumors. Your situation may, in addition, have unique potential problems.

S T R O K E

♦ **1 What was the type of stroke I had?**

Stroke is a general term indicating that an area of brain has been permanently damaged. Damage may result from blocking of a blood vessel to the area, bursting of a blood vessel with bleeding into the area, or a number of less common conditions. Knowing the specific cause helps direct future therapy.

♦ **2 Are special studies needed to find the cause? What steps should be taken to prevent future strokes or transient loss of function?**

Once the type of stroke has been determined, special studies may be needed to further clarify cause and determine risk of future events. For example, if a piece of clot broke off from somewhere and traveled to the brain, attempts will be made to find the source of the clot and to prevent further pieces breaking off. If a stroke was precipitated by high blood pressure, attempts will be made to better control the pressure.

◆ 3 Can I benefit from medication?

There are many roles for medication in stroke patients which range from control of high blood pressure to prevention of seizures as a complication of stroke. You may be someone who would benefit, depending on the cause of your stroke, your disability, and other factors.

◆ 4 If surgery is recommended, what are the risks?

Occasionally a stroke victim will have a problem that is amenable to surgery, but these surgical procedures also often have high risks. If surgery is proposed for you, be sure you understand fully the risks and chance of benefit before undertaking it.

◆ 5 What are my chances of regaining strength in the affected limbs and/or speech if it is impaired?

While no one can answer this question precisely, certain factors predict a favorable outcome, others an unfavorable outcome. Even with the predictive factors, the chances of recovery depend, to some degree, on the patient's motivation and whether or not poststroke complications occur.

◆ 6 What physical (and speech) rehabilitation is available for me? And how long should I have rehabilitation therapy?

Nearly all hospitals have programs of rehabilitation for victims of strokes, since it is a common illness inflicting usually severe disability on the victim. The length of time rehabilitation therapy should be continued depends on many factors like original disability, whether or not the patient is responding to rehabilitation measures, and the motivation of the patient.

◆ **7   Are home physical therapy programs available, and can my spouse (or other relative) be trained to help me with this?**

Transportation to outpatient physical therapy may be difficult, and inpatient therapy is often limited in time and also quite expensive. Home programs are often desirable and effective and may be available in your area.

◆ **8   What are possible sources of funding for a rehabilitation program for me?**

Your doctor, the social services representative in your hospital, as well as the local chapter of the Stroke Recovery Association may be able to suggest sources of funding to pay for rehabilitation services. Insurance policies may cover certain types of rehabilitation as well.

◆ **9   Can you suggest any equipment (and where to buy it) that I could get to make my home care easier?**

Stroke victims often have major adaptations to make when they go home. They may not be able to walk or, if so, only with aids like metal walkers. Navigating stairs may be impossible. Equipment to aid in getting into a bathtub, wheelchairs, commodes, special beds, and so on may be useful in helping the patient adjust at home.

◆ **10   Are home nursing services available to assist our family on a temporary or permanent basis?**

Stroke patients may have difficulties in eating, bowel and bladder control, taking medications, and other areas of daily living. Home nursing care is often available on at least a temporary basis through government or other agencies.

◆ **11   Are there complications of stroke I should be on the lookout for?**

There is the potential for many complications whenever part of the body is not functioning normally. In the case of strokes, the risk of complications varies with the areas affected, the amount of paralysis, underlying medical conditions, and so on. Complications can include pneumonia, seizures, contractions, loss of mobility of affected limbs, and pain in affected limbs.

◆ **12   Is there a branch of the Stroke Recovery Association in this area?**

Associations to help stroke victims will have information about many of the services that you will need. However, in addition, they will be able to provide another service, which is invaluable to many families: that is, you will be able to talk to other patients and families who are facing the same problems and disabilities and discuss how they are handling them. In Canada the Heart Foundation has information for stroke patients.

ULCER DISEASE

◆ **1   Where is my ulcer located, and what is the likely cause?**

Ulcers may be located in the stomach or upper intestine (duodenum). These locations have different implications regarding cause, potential for healing and recurrence, potential for becoming or being cancerous, and so on. Sometimes, a likely cause, including anything from a medication to a genetic disease, can be identified, but often not.

◆ **2   What sort of studies will I need to evaluate my ulcer?**

Often ulcers are diagnosed by x-ray studies but if these are inconclusive, if the ulcer is in the stomach, or in a variety of other situations, an endoscopy may be recommended in which the ulcer can be directly visualized through a tube placed through the mouth and esophagus into the stomach.

◆ **3   Should I have biopsies taken to rule out cancer?**

Some ulcers have a location or appearance where risk of cancer, particularly in older age groups, is quite high.

Biopsy (taking small pieces of tissue) can be done quite easily by placing a tube through the mouth and esophagus into the stomach (endoscopy).

♦ **4   Can other medical problems or drugs have a role in causing the ulcer or impairing healing?**

A number of drugs affect the stomach lining and may predispose to ulcer formation. Other medical conditions (e.g., lung disease in smokers as well as smoking itself or illnesses with high serum calcium) sometimes are also associated with increased incidence of ulcers.

♦ **5   Can I improve healing by making any changes in my life-style?**

Sometimes stress or personality characteristics may play a role in the formation of an ulcer. Smoking has already been mentioned as a contributing factor. Heavy intake of aspirin is a risk factor. Other individual factors may also come into play and should be discussed with the doctor.

♦ **6   How do I take my medications, and what side effects should I watch for?**

A number of medications are now available to assist or promote healing of ulcers. Timing of medications may be important, including when taken in relationship to meals. Also, certain unique patient factors, e.g., age, may predispose to some of the medications' side effects.

♦ **7   Will my ulcer medications interact with the medications I am taking for other illness? What dosage adjustments are needed?**

Especially the newer histamine blocking agents are known to influence the blood level of many other drugs. To avoid serious problems from these drugs, the dosages may have to be adjusted.

♦ **8   Will I need follow-up investigations to monitor for healing?**

Failure to heal may be suggestive of malignancy (cancer) in some types of ulcer. In others, this may be rare. Other factors may indicate a need for further investigations to check healing.

◆ 9 How long should it take for healing to occur?

Again, your ulcer may differ from your neighbor's in the time it takes to heal. Yours may be in a different location, you may have other predisposing factors, you may not respond to medication as well, etc., and your expected healing time might be quite different.

◆ 10 What are the chances it will recur?

Whether the predisposing factors can be identified and modified will influence the answer to this question. Other factors might include location of ulcer, personal characteristics, speed of healing.

◆ 11 Does diet have any influence on my ulcer disease, and should I have a special diet?

The role of diet is not felt to be as important in ulcer disease as it once was, but the issue is not settled. You may have a specific situation in which following a particular diet or at least avoiding specific foods is desirable.

◆ 12 Should I avoid any types of antacids?

Antacids are a common means of treating ulcer disease, and many are available over the counter at drugstores. However, they are not all the same in composition, and some may be dangerous or undesirable if you have certain other medical problems. Also, some may be more effective than others for you.

◆ 13 Should I be on the lookout for signs of bleeding?

The underlying factors relating to your ulcer disease, previous history, and many other things may play a role in whether or not bleeding or perforation of the ulcer is likely to occur. While the doctor certainly will not be able to predict this, if he has reason to be concerned in your case, he will tell you what to watch for.

◆ 14 Under what circumstances would surgery be considered in my treatment?

Many unique factors enter into a question of surgical intervention. These might include amount of bleeding, ability to stop bleeding, recurrence of bleeding, medical problems that might complicate surgery, and many others. It may be best to find out the circumstances you might be facing if bleeding occurred. Occasionally, there may be indications other than bleeding for surgery in ulcer disease.

◆ 15 If I think I am bleeding or my pain gets worse, what should I do?

It is always best to have a clear-cut plan of action to follow before an emergency occurs. Find out whom to call, where to go, and what measures to take on your own if you get into this situation.

◆ 16 Are there alternative medications if I cannot tolerate what I am taking?

There are now a number of different categories of drugs available for ulcer therapy. If one or two types of drugs are not successful or tolerated, an alternate can be tried that may be better tolerated.

◆ 17 Are the drugs I am taking safe if I should become pregnant?

Ulcers can well occur in women of childbearing age. If pregnancy is planned, determine what is known about the safety of drugs you are taking. If the safety is uncertain, it may be best to delay pregnancy until the ulcer is healed.

♦

UNDERSTANDING
MEDICATIONS

♦

Drugs or medications, of which there are thousands, are a very pervasive and expensive part of medical practice in North America. We have come to believe that if we are just given the right pill, we will be cured. This, of course, is nonsense. Most of the medications that are available do not cure at all, but rather ameliorate symptoms, alter mood, or slow progression of disease, hopefully to a degree that will help us live our lives more fully. Relieving symptoms allows us to decrease the time spent dwelling on them—be it pain, anxiety, or difficulty breathing—and allows us to use our time in more fruitful ways.

To be able to use your medications to their best advantage, you must become sophisticated about the drugs that are being recommended for you. Only when you learn the potential risks, benefits, strengths, and limitations of the medications available for you will you and your doctor be able to set up and manipulate a drug program and dosing schedule that will provide maximum reduction in symptoms or, when possible, a cure.

Several sources of information about drugs are available. The American Medical Association has prepared drug information sheets for patients on about one hundred commonly used drugs. These are written in easy to understand terms and provide information about interactions with other medications, as well as side effects and toxic effects of the drugs. Similar information can be obtained from the American Academy of Family Physicians and from the Pharmacy Service of the American Association of Retired Persons. An updated book with drug information written for lay persons is published by the United States Pharmacopeal (USP) Convention, Inc. It is called *Advice for the Patient.* Some of these sources charge a small fee for their information; others do not. The addresses and telephone numbers of these sources are listed at the end of this section.

In recent years, a number of books simplifying the terminology have been published for laymen. These can be found in libraries and bookstores.

More sophisticated and complete information is contained in the *Physician's Desk Reference (PDR)* in the United States or the *Compendium of Pharmaceuticals and Specialties* (*CPS*) in Canada. These give the drug company's description and formula of the drug, the indications for the drug, and the contraindications (or situations in which the drug should *not* be used), as well as reported side effects, toxic effects, usual dosages, and uses for which the medications are available. One section of the *PDR* and *CPS* also shows pictures of most drugs that are included in the book so that you can visually verify the drug you have. Also available is a supplement to the *PDR* which lists over-the-counter or nonprescription drugs in the same way in which the main publication lists prescription drugs.

A few precautions must be followed in using any of these books which are available in most libraries and are reissued in updated form each year.

First, since the *PDR* and *CPS* are published for doctors, they are written in technical terms and may be difficult to understand.

Second, you may be given a drug for a reason that is not listed in the indications. The *PDR* lists indications for which the government has approved the drug. Many times new areas will be found in which drugs are helpful (such as the beneficial effect of antiinflammatory, antiarthritic drugs on premenstrual cramps), but it will take several years for the government to approve this as an indication.

Third, contraindications may be general rules, but in a case where a particular patient really needs a drug for disease control—in a life-threatening illness, for example—the doctor may feel that the potential benefit justifies the drug's use in spite of considerable risk. (This should always be explained in advance to the patient.)

Fourth, all side effects or adverse reactions ever reported in persons using the drugs are listed in these books, even if they occurred in only one person or if the relationship of side effects to the drug was never proven. Thus, when you read the list of side effects for any drug listed, it may seem appalling. Since, in general, the possible benefits to you of a particular drug usually far outweigh these risks, the adverse reactions should be read in that light. For example, the list of adverse reactions to ampicillin—a penicillin derivative and one of the most commonly prescribed antibiotics—includes, in addition to rashes and other common allergic reactions, diarrhea and colitis, liver effects, and six different effects on the blood components.

Finally, the recommended dosages listed may have been modified for your particular problem from those listed in these references, because of some other complicating medical conditions or more current recommendations in the medical literature.

The *Merck Manual* is another source listing many drugs with information similar to the *PDR*. This also is geared toward the medical profession and uses medical terminology.

Certainly, valuable information can be gained from these sources and be useful supplementation to what your doctor tells you. However, the best, most personalized and useful information comes by asking your doctor the right questions, because that information will be tailored to your unique situation.

Addresses for the aforementioned information services follow:

1. AMERICAN ACADEMY OF FAMILY PHYSICIANS
   600 Maryland Avenue, SW
   Suite 700
   Washington, DC 20024
   (202) 488-7448

2. MEDICATION INSTRUCTION LEAFLETS FOR SENIORS
   American Association of Retired Persons
   Retired Persons Services Branch
   One Prince Street
   Alexandria, VA 22314
   (703) 684-0244

3. AMERICAN MEDICAL ASSOCIATION
   Attention: Order Department
   535 N. Dearborn Street
   Chicago, IL 60610
   (312) 380-7268

4. COMPENDIUM OF PHARMACEUTICALS AND SPE-
   CIALTIES
   Canadian Pharmaceutical Association
   101–1815 Alta Vista Drive
   Ottawa, Ontario
   Canada K1G 3Y6

5. PHYSICIAN'S DESK REFERENCE
   Medical Economics Company, Inc.
   Oradell, NJ 07649

6. UNITED STATES PHARMACOPEAL CONVENTION,
   INC.
   12601 Twin Brook Pkwy.
   Rockville, MD 20852

The following list of questions should give you a good
understanding of the drugs, what you can expect from
them, and how you can utilize them. The first set of
questions give you important information about the
role of drugs in your particular illness and the second
set give information about the drugs themselves.

THE ROLE OF DRUGS IN THE ILLNESS

◆ 1 **What types of drugs are used in this disease, and
how do they work?**

It will help you to understand your illness if you find out
how medications work. This is called the *mechanism of
action.* Most doctors are happy to have a patient show
that much interest and can sit down and explain the
basic concepts quite simply.

   Do the drugs alter a basic mechanism of the disease?
Do they simply change a consequence of the underlying
disease? Do they not affect the disease process at all,
but rather influence one's perception of it?

   For example, in rheumatoid arthritis, the pain medications usually work by reducing inflammation; in other

situations—say, after an operation—where relief of pain is important, but inflammation is not the cause, the drugs used may act by altering one's perception of the pain.

Different sorts of drugs may be available that work at different steps in the disease process. Sometimes, these drugs can effectively be used in combination. In congestive heart failure, diuretics reduce the accumulation of excess body fluid which is secondary to poor heart function; digoxin works directly to improve the contraction process of the heart. The two often can be used effectively in combination.

♦ 2   Why are you choosing these particular drugs for me?

Often multiple drugs are available to treat an illness. You may know other persons with the same illness who are receiving completely different drugs!

What medications are chosen depends on the particular characteristics of the patient, the manifestations of the illness in the patient, and the experience and comfort of the doctor with certain drugs. It will help you to know what factors have been considered in your particular situation, to improve your understanding of the approach and why it is the best approach for you.

Also, often drugs with similar actions are provided by several different companies and, therefore, have different brand names. Ask if you can get the generic form of a drug, which is often much cheaper.

Here is an example of varying therapies. You and your neighbor both have high blood pressure. You have been given Dyazide and Inderal for control, but she is receiving Hygroton and Aldomet. Both Dyazide and Hygroton are diuretics or "water pills." You receive Dyazide because you have problems with low blood potassium and this drug is potassium-sparing; she does not require this feature. You receive, in addition, Inderal and cannot tolerate Aldomet because of a history of rash thought to be caused by Aldomet. Your neighbor tolerates Aldomet well, but cannot take Inderal because it worsens her asthma.

◆ 3 Do the drugs I am receiving cure this illness?

While a few diseases are curable by drug therapy, e.g., infections, many of them are not, and the drugs are used for a variety of other reasons. Be clear about the role of the drugs you are using (see question 4), and do not harbor misconceptions about "cures," since this may lead you to quit taking or inadequately take or abuse drugs which can be quite important to your therapy and in large dosages may be quite toxic.

◆ 4 If the drugs do not cure my illness, what effect should I expect from them?

Drugs can be used for a variety of purposes in illness, particularly chronic illness for which there is no known cure. Some of the common uses are as follows:

a. Improvement of symptoms, as in medications given for heart failure or for prevention of angina pectoris (the pain usually caused by atherosclerotic heart vessels which prevent adequate blood flow to the heart muscle when there is an increased demand for oxygen).

b. Arresting the progression of disease, as the use of chemotherapeutic agents in cancer. In many cases, it is known the drugs are unlikely to cure the illness, but may temporarily arrest the tumor growth and give the patient some months or years of productive life.

c. Prevention of damage to other organs. Drugs used to control high blood pressure aim to prevent the eventual destructive effects of many years of high pressure on various organs. Specifically, the risk of strokes, kidney disease, and heart attacks can be markedly reduced by the use of medications in this disease.

d. Prevention of recurrence of symptoms. Among the most common drugs used for this are many asthma drugs which are designed to be used continuously when the patient is feeling well and, when so used, prevent most acute attacks of wheezing.

Once you understand how medications are supposed to function in your disease, it will be easier for you to discuss with your doctor any problems that arise with the medication or how well the medication is fulfilling the purpose for which it is intended.

♦ 5 How long will I have to take medication?

Infections, luckily, often require only a few days of treatment; high blood pressure must be treated for life. The duration of drug therapy ranges from one dose to usage for life, depending upon the illness. Your physician may or may not know how long you will require medications. Many times treatment is pragmatic and will be adjusted according to the patient's needs and responses. At least you will be able to get an idea of the course of therapy by asking.

♦ 6 Can you give me a plan for what we will do if this treatment doesn't work?

If you have a general idea of what might be coming up if your treatment fails, *or* if your treatment is known to be useful only for a certain phase of the illness, *or* if the amount of drug you can take is limited because of toxicity, etc., you will feel more in control of your situation. You may not know exactly what your future will hold, but having a general idea of the possibilities will ease your mind some and disperse some of the anxiety and fear of the unknown.

THE DRUGS THEMSELVES

♦ 1 What is the dosing interval?

Drug dosing interval—how often you have to take the drug—is based on the half-life of the drug and may vary from once a month (some injections) to four or more times a day. In the past few years, many drugs have been formulated in slow-release forms so that the pill or capsule can be taken less often, usually once or twice a day, to get the same effect. Check to see if you can take your medication in this form because it is much simpler to take fewer pills once or twice a day. If you have several types of medication to take, small boxes with multiple compartments are available. Each morning you put whatever drugs you need for that day in its proper compartment. This way, if you can't remember whether you have taken your drugs, if the pills for a particular dosing time are gone, then you will know you have taken them.

♦ 2   **Are there any particular rules for taking the drugs?**

Sometimes drugs are more easily tolerated or work better if taken in a certain order, e.g., the various inhalers used in asthma. Other rules might involve means of administration—e.g., whether the drug should be swallowed whole or chewed, placed under the tongue or swallowed, taken with food in the stomach or without, with other medications or not.

♦ 3   **Are there interactions with other drugs, foods, sunlight, or alcohol?**

This is a *critical* question. Many drugs have interactions, usually because they are broken down and removed by the same systems in the body, especially the liver and kidneys. In the liver, a drug can either induce (speed up degradation by) enzymes or compete for the same enzyme degradation with other drugs. Thus, taking one drug may either decrease another drug to inadequate blood levels or increase it to toxic blood levels, depending on its effects on the liver. Cimetidine (Tagamet) taken for ulcer disease may interfere with degradation of theophylline (e.g., Theo-Dur) taken for asthma and therefore increase theophylline to toxic blood levels. Warfarin, a blood thinner (anticoagulant), interacts with many drugs, and the interactions can result in risk of either excessive bleeding or excessive clot formation.

Food may also be a problem. Taking the drug with food may interfere with absorption. In other circumstances, drugs should be taken with food. Tetracycline is a chelator and, therefore, is inactivated if taken with calcium-containing foods, since it binds with the calcium. It, as well as a number of other compounds, can sensitize the skin to sunlight, and sunscreens must be worn when taking those compounds. Alcohol may cause vomiting when taken with some drugs and, since it has effects on the liver, may also influence the elimination of drugs. The kidney most often influences drug dosages when kidney function is impaired, thereby reducing elimination of the drug.

◆ 4   What are the side effects of this drug?

Toxic effects are effects which may be harmful to you and are a subset of side effects. Side effects include, in addition to toxic effects, anything caused by the drug that may be annoying (or may be unpleasant), but which is not dangerous. Toxic effects are often caused by excessive amounts of drug. Side effects need not be.

As mentioned at the beginning of this chapter, the *PDR* lists all the side effects ever reported for a drug. Find out from your doctor what the most important and most common are, how to look for them, and exactly how often they occur. Also, you should establish if you, for any reason, are particularly apt to develop side effects.

◆ 5   What are the toxic effects?

Be sure to clarify what the dangerous side effects are, how common they are, and if you are in a high-risk group and how you recognize it. Consider isoniazid. It is an excellent drug to treat tuberculosis. Unfortunately, it has a serious side effect, drug-induced hepatitis. This is uncommon under the age 35, but becomes increasingly common as a person ages. It is heralded by pain over the liver, nausea, and loss of appetite. If it is noted early and the drug stopped, the patient nearly always recovers. A minor degree of hepatitis is not uncommon with this drug, but it is a toxic effect in only a small number of cases. In this situation, the toxicity need not be dose-related.

♦ 6 **Is there a wide gap between toxic and therapeutic amounts of this drug?**

Overdosage is always a problem when medication is prescribed. Some drugs have a very narrow range between toxic effects and the amounts necessary for a therapeutic affect; in others this difference may be large and, therefore, risk of toxicity small. With some medications, for example, just doubling your dose may cause toxic symptoms.

♦ 7 **If someone accidentally takes my drug, or I accidentally take too many, what is the best course of action?**

Find out the telephone number of your poison control center and keep it on hand. Is this a medicine that must be removed from the stomach as soon as possible? Does it require more drastic approaches if overdosing occurs?

♦ 8 **Are there any long-term adverse effects?**

With certain drugs, such as anticancer agents, effects of the drugs can become apparent many years from the time they were taken. For example, certain chemotherapeutic drugs seem to predispose to new cancers, which may arise years after their use. Also, these drugs may result many years later in sterility.

Another situation where one should be concerned about long-term effects is when the drug is taken for a long period of time, usually years. For example, steroids may have many untoward effects, especially when taken for long periods of time.

♦ 9 **Can I take generic drugs?**

Drugs can be very expensive, especially if they must be taken for a long time. Many of the commonly used drugs are available as generic (nonbrand-name) compounds and cost much less that way. Prescriptions can be written using the generic name for the drug, and usually a box on the prescription form states that a generic compound may be used. Request this from the doctor and the pharmacist. Occasionally, there is a reason for using a specific brand-name drug. Ask your doctor to explain the situation to you.

♦ **10   Is there any other way to reduce the expense of taking this drug?**

As mentioned, medications are often very expensive, and they are not covered under most insurance plans. The cost may be a hardship for you. Sometimes an alternative drug or formulation, say, a different antibiotic, can be substituted at reduced cost. Sometimes, a different dosing schedule with less use of the drug but more effort on your part will be an acceptable alternative. Other creative ways to reduce cost may be worked out by you and your doctor.

♦ **11   What if I become pregnant while taking the drug?**

Generally speaking, doctors agree that it is unwise to take drugs during pregnancy, and nearly all drugs carry a warning that the drug has not been shown to be safe in pregnant women; studies have not been done to clearly demonstrate safety. Practically speaking, some women have illnesses, like high blood pressure or epilepsy, where drugs must be continued throughout pregnancy. Only in a few cases have drugs been shown to clearly increase the likelihood of malformation and/or miscarriages. However, if you are taking one of the drugs with which there is a known risk of fetal malformations, you should be aware in order to make the best decision for you.

♦ **12   Does this drug interfere with sex in any way?**

This may be a difficult question to ask, but it is important, particularly for men, since a number of medications, e.g., some of the drugs used for the very common disease high blood pressure, can prevent a man from being able to achieve an erection or cause other types of sexual dysfunction. This type of problem can usually be alleviated by changing the drugs.

◆ 13 Do the medications cause sterility?

This is a very important consideration, primarily in the use of cancer chemotherapy. The use of such drugs is not undertaken lightly, and if they are suggested, they are probably the only effective drugs for the disease. Men have the option in such situations to "bank" semen, which can be frozen for future use.

◆ 14 Can the drug be stopped suddenly or doses missed without any ill effects?

Most medications can be stopped without any dangerous side effects. However, a few drugs when stopped suddenly may have serious implications for your body. These can include such diverse problems as leaving the body without adequate responses to stress (as in the case of corticosteroids) to a rebound occurrence of the original condition (as in the case of some antihigh-blood-pressure medicines). In these cases, you often have to taper the dosage of the drug over time. Get a tapering schedule from your doctor should this cessation of drug become necessary. Also, if you are taking such a drug, keep an extra prescription on hand in the event you lose your pills.

◆ 15 What should I do if I suffer a side effect of a drug?

Usually your doctor will instruct you to call him if a side or toxic effect of a drug occurs. He may instruct you to immediately discontinue the drug if certain effects develop; on the other hand, some side effects are so common and mild, he will usually warn you about them and ask you not to call unless they are unnecessarily bothersome. Clarify this issue with the physician at the outset to decrease your level of anxiety as well as limit the number of phone calls to the doctor.

Compliance with medications is critical to effective treatment of many illnesses. Often failure of patients to take medications reflects more their lack of understanding of the instructions for taking the medicines and their ignorance of potential, often minor side effects than it does their unwillingness to take drugs. If the drugs that are useful for your illness are reviewed for you according to the suggestions made here, they will become familiar friends rather than distrusted intruders and hopefully you will ultimately benefit from their proper use.

CHAPTER FIVE

♦

UNDERSTANDING
PROCEDURES
AND TESTS

♦

It seems almost impossible to visit a doctor anymore without being subjected to a series of tests. Gone are the days when diagnoses were made solely on the basis of history and physical exam—but so are many of the missed diagnoses, ill-advised therapies, and early deaths. Now the doctor tries to use pertinent historical and examination data to order appropriate confirmatory tests. Using the patient's symptoms and examination findings to guide one in the ordering of the most useful laboratory studies is an art that is difficult for many doctors to master. Thus, often more tests than are absolutely needed may be ordered. Combine this with patients who are understandably reluctant about undergoing extensive, time-consuming, privacy-invading studies, some with serious potential complications, and you have uncovered a big area for potential breakdown of communication between patient and doctor.

This chapter is an attempt to lessen your fear of tests by understanding the tests as well as what they are expected to measure or evaluate. First I will give you some general information about different types of tests. This is followed by a series of questions through which you can gain specific information about the tests under consideration for you, and whether or not they may really be indicated.

In the evaluation of the symptoms that you present, laboratory tests may serve several purposes. The first, and most obvious, is to assist in making the diagnosis. Just as important though, they establish "baseline" values for you. These can be especially important if you are being started on therapy that may alter these values.

The tests might be used either to monitor the success or failure of therapy or to pick up early complications. As an example, let's take a very simple test: the measurement of the number and kinds of white blood cells from a small blood sample. These two measurements from a simple test can be used to support the diagnosis of leukemias or infections or to monitor the success of treatment of either of these. In other situations, the same measurements can be used to detect a complication of therapy, bone marrow suppression.

Different patients with the same illness will not necessarily undergo the same tests, because each patient's manifestations of a disease may be quite unique. In one person a single test may make the diagnosis; in another, several tests may be required. The order in which tests are done may also differ. This depends on several factors, including the facilities available where you are being evaluated, how familiar the doctor is with using the different tests, the doctor's experience with reliability of the tests in his institution, and so on. In general, the doctor will try to balance the risks and yields. Since often the most likely tests to yield a diagnosis (e.g., a surgical biopsy) are also the most costly, and have the most risk, the doctor may well first order a test that is a bit less likely to give a definite diagnosis, but is also less dangerous. If the diagnosis is made, so much the better. If not, he can move on to the riskier but potentially higher yield test.

Another way to categorize tests, which often corresponds basically to the risk-yield categorization just described, is noninvasive vs. invasive. These terms are frequently used by doctors in describing tests. The terms are quite accurately descriptive in that the less invasive a test is, the less actual violation of body space occurs. Thus, a simple chest x-ray would be *noninvasive* and may point out an abnormality but not give a specific diagnosis. However, the patient might have to go as far as having a piece of lung surgically removed under general anesthesia to make the actual diagnosis. This *invasive* procedure will be diagnostic but carries the risks of anesthesia, postoperative infections, and at least several days of pain. The patient will be left with a scar, possibly have persistent pain, and incur time lost from work.

To better familiarize you with the more commonly ordered tests, following are general descriptions.

BLOOD TESTS / TESTS ON BODY FLUID COLLECTIONS

Blood tests are the most common of tests done on body fluids. Most often blood is collected from a vein near the elbow. This procedure is called venipuncture. The discomfort is mainly from the prick of the needle, and the risks are minimal. Occasionally some bleeding will occur under the skin which leaves a bruise (hematoma). (This may not be attractive but causes no long-term damage.) Blood can also be taken from arteries. This is called arterial puncture and is necessary to measure the oxygen and carbon dioxide levels in the blood. Unfortunately, the pain associated with it is somewhat greater than that of a venipuncture and is described as throbbing.

Studies that yield important information can be done on any body fluid. Collection of some, like urine or sputum, is simple and without risk. To collect fluid from within the chest (pleural fluid), from around the heart (pericardial fluid), from within the abdomen (ascitic fluid), from within the spinal canal (spinal fluid), from within joint spaces, or in pregnant women from within the womb (amniotic fluid) requires blindly placing a needle into an area where the fluid is. This involves the discomfort of the needle stick and occasional pain from other structures through which the needle is passed and has more associated risk than collecting blood, sputum, or urine. Be sure you fully understand the risks involved in these collections.

ECG, EMG, EEG

These studies measure the electrical activity in the heart (electrocardiography, ECG or EKG), muscle (electromyography, EMG), and brain (electroencephalography, EEG). Normal patterns are known and abnormal patterns can be recognized. The measuring is done by placing electrodes on the skin (for ECG and EEG) or in the muscle (for EMG, which also involves the discomfort of placing small needles into the muscle). There are essentially no risks to these tests, since they merely record electrical activity.

ULTRASOUND (SONOGRAPHY) OR ECHOGRAMS

These are studies in which sound waves are bounced off body structures beneath the skin, and the "echoes" are electrically transduced and displayed as a picture on a small screen. A small "microphone" is placed over the organ or area to be evaluated. Since different densities of tissue (e.g., blood, fluids, fat, bone muscles, tissue) reflect back different amounts of the sound, they send back different echoes. The organ shapes and sizes can be recorded, and when these differ from known normal patterns, diseases may be suggested. These tests can be used to delineate nearly every body organ. No side effects from these studies have been noted and no risks are known. Yet uses of these tests are many—from location of abnormal accumulation of fluids, to diagnosis, to monitoring of function or treatment.

X-RAYS, CT SCANS, TOMOGRAMS, FLUOROSCOPIC X-RAYS

X-rays, computerized tomographic (CT) scans, and tomograms all are tests in which beams of radiation are passed through body structures. Again, different densities of tissue absorb different amounts of radiation (the denser, the more absorption), and what isn't absorbed passes through the tissue and exposes a film, just like light beams expose a film in a camera. Thus, bones, fat, and organs all appear a different shade of gray on an x-ray. Some x-ray studies include the use of special substances to better picture the part of the body that is being studied. Gastrointestinal studies use barium as an enema or swallowed to outline the different structures of the gut. Kidney x-rays often require the use of a dye that is opaque (absorbs x-rays) to outline the organs adequately, as does visualization of the gallbladder.

If a routine x-ray can be considered a photograph of part of the body, fluoroscopy is a movie. That is, it is a dynamic x-ray picture of the movements and functions of parts of the body that are being studied. When gastrointestinal studies are being done, the movement of barium, e.g., is watched under a fluoroscopy machine. In many of the endoscopic procedures (see later in this chapter), fluoroscopic visualization of the organs being studied aids in correct positioning of the endoscope, biopsy tools, etc.

CT scans and tomograms are particular types of x-rays in which special techniques are used to make more precise pictures of certain areas. CT scans take pictures of "slices" of the body. In a usual x-ray, the person sits or lies in front of a piece of film. Then a small amount of radiation is passed through the person and that which is not absorbed exposes the film. In a CT scan, the person lies on a table which moves through the x-ray mechanism, a large donut-shaped structure. Generally, a centimeter-wide slice of the person is filmed, then the table is advanced to the next "cut." Radiation signals are transformed by computer into a picture which shows internal structures. By looking at a series of these pictures (or slices), each of which covers about 1 cm of body height, doctors can get a three-dimensional view of the part of the body in which they are interested. Tomograms are simply a type of x-ray in which the x-ray beam is shot from different angles, focused on a particular area in the body. The idea is to blur out surrounding structures in order to get a better view of a particular abnormality usually noted on a routine x-ray.

Risks of x-rays are really two. The first is radiation. The amount of radiation is generally very small in an x-ray. It does vary from one type of x-ray to another, and radiation damage can be cumulative. Even so, it would take a great many x-ray studies to put you in danger of any serious side effects. To fetuses, however, the risk is not clear. Childbearing-age women should have the abdomen lead-shielded when x-rays are done on other areas and have x-rays only when absolutely necessary if they are pregnant.

The second risk applies to those studies in which a radiopaque dye (a dye that absorbs radiation and is therefore highly visible) is used. This dye is used in many x-ray studies and in CT scans. It is injected into a vein just before the study and outlines blood vessels and urine-containing structures. This dye can give the person a hot flushed sensation, which, though unpleasant, usually passes quickly without ill effect. However, the dye can trigger an allergic response in some patients. This can cause anything from a rash to a sudden loss of blood pressure, and can be quite serious. It is impossible to predict and if it has ever happened to a person, future dye studies should be avoided if possible. If they are absolutely necessary, the patient should have drugs ahead of time to try to prevent a similar reaction. Dyes can also further impair kidney function in patients who have some underlying kidney disease.

MRI (MAGNETIC RESONANCE IMAGING)

The latest technique developed to look into and outline organs in the body is magnetic resonance imaging. The picture produced looks much like that of a CT scan, but no radiation is used. The patient lies on a table which is surrounded by a large donut-shaped magnet. As the body passes through the magnet, the charged hydrogen atoms in the body align momentarily with the powerful external magnet, then flip back into their own magnetic field. These "flips" generate a radiowave-like signal. Since the hydrogen atoms in different organs give off different frequency signals, a computer can then translate the different radio signals into pictures. The exact role of this machine has not been established because of its newness. So far, side effects have not been seen.

NUCLEAR SCANS

Nuclear scans are another common type of test which uses small amounts of radiation to outline organs and abnormalities in organs. Elements—gallium, thallium, technetium, and some others—are made radioactive by bombardment in a nuclear accelerator. These are then tagged to molecules that are found in the body, like albumin, and placed in a liquid which can be injected into the body. Depending upon the element, and what it is tagged to, it will tend to collect in certain organs that are "avid" for these substances. Sometimes abnormalities are "hot" spots (accumulate excessive element), others are "cold" spots (collect little or no radioactive material), depending on the organ and the pathological damage being assessed and the element used.

To do these tests, the patient first receives an injection of the radioactive material in a vein. Then one waits a period of time, which may vary from a few minutes to one or two days, depending on the organ being evaluated and the material used. When sufficient radioactive material has accumulated in the organ by being picked up from the bloodstream, a camera or scanner is used to make the picture. This scanner is a large round machine which looks something like a bass drum. Depending upon what is being scanned, it may be placed over, under or beside the patient, who may be lying or sitting. The scanner actually records radioactivity given off by the trapped radioactive element and appears on the scan as a mass of tiny dots.

Risks of nuclear scans are very tiny. The small amount of radioactive material in you is usually gone in a few hours and at most in a few days. It is not a danger to those around you. One word of caution, again, is that the effect on developing fetuses is not clear, so nuclear scans should be avoided in pregnant women unless absolutely necessary.

FIBEROPTIC ENDOSCOPIC PROCEDURES

With the advent of fiberoptic technology, a whole new group of important studies became available both for diagnosis and for instituting and following therapy. Fiberoptics is the technique of transmitting light along flexible plastic fibers so that a light source at one end can result in bright illumination of the other end of the fiber which is several inches to several feet away. By using a set of lenses, a person looking down the fibers at the same end as the light source can visualize structures at the far end. Since these fibers are flexible, the operator can maneuver the tube through and around nearly every opening in the human body without impairing his visualization of whatever is at the far end of the fibers. Fiberoptic endoscopy is the term given to any procedure in which this technology is used to "look into" any of the body's hollow organs.

That means the doctor can actually see a stomach ulcer, a lung cancer, or a polyp in the colon. Today, fiberoptic procedures are done in most hospitals and some doctors' offices. Esophagoscopy and gastroscopy involve going through the mouth and down the throat to look at the esophagus and stomach. Colonoscopy and sigmoidoscopy are done through the anus to look at the large bowel. Bronchoscopy is the technique used to look into the airways of the lung by entering either through the mouth or nose, then passing through the vocal cords to gain a view of the airways. Specialized diagnostic or therapeutic techniques can be done during these procedures. These include biopsies, laser treatment, and a number of special techniques related to each organ.

Most fiberoptic endoscopies are done with local anesthesia similar to that used in a dentist's office. Before the procedure, the patient is often given an injection designed to relax him and in some cases to dry up secretions. The patient will either lie or sit for the procedure. Often a teaching apparatus is available so the patient can participate in the procedure if he wishes.

Risks from these procedures are generally small. There is a small risk of reactions from the local anesthesia, but the greater risks are from complications when pieces of tissue (biopsies) are obtained. These risks include bleeding and perforation of the organ which, though rare, are potentially serious. Make sure the risks are carefully explained to you before the procedure.

BIOPSIES

Biopsy is the taking of an actual piece of tissue so it can be cultured or looked at under a microscope to make an exact diagnosis. Biopsies can be taken from almost any organ or part of the body. These are considered invasive tests and therefore are somewhat more risky.

If the biopsy is done with direct visualization of the organ, it is called an open biopsy. This often requires general anesthesia and is a type of surgery. The piece of tissue obtained will be large and therefore should be adequate to make a diagnosis. Bleeding can be surgically controlled. The risks are those related to anesthesia and surgery. Reactions to drugs, wound infections, and pneumonia are all potential complications. Of course, there is considerable pain and often at least several days of hospital stay. If the organ lies just beneath the skin and not in a body cavity, e.g., some lymph nodes, of course the risks and discomfort are much less.

The other type of biopsy is the closed biopsy, in which pieces of tissue are obtained usually by placing a hollow needle through the skin (called percutaneous) into the organ to be sampled without directly visualizing the organ. The advantages to this approach are that it is easier and less painful for the patient, it can be done under local anesthesia, and it usually yields a large enough sample to make a diagnosis. The disadvantages are that (1) since the target is not seen, it can be missed; (2) there may not be enough tissue obtained for diagnosis, so the test is in vain; and (3) unrecognized bleeding may occur since the biopsy site is not visible. This last complication, however, is always carefully monitored for. Organs often approached by closed biopsy include liver, bone marrow, kidney, lung, prostate, and pleura (the covering of the lung). Sometimes this type of biopsy is done with the aid of CT scan or ultrasound to better locate organs and be more certain of obtaining a good specimen.

CATHETERIZATION OF BLOOD VESSELS

Angiograms and venograms are tests in which a hollow tube (catheter) is placed into a blood vessel. In angiograms an artery is entered, and in venograms a vein. The catheter is usually placed in the best position to see the organ to be studied. Then a dye that shows up under x-ray is put through the catheter and outlines the vessels just beyond the end of the catheter. If the vessels that are seen when filled with the dye are abnormal in shape or configuration, if they are being pushed out of their normal distribution, if the dye lies outside the vessels, etc., the doctor can be alerted to a variety of diseases. Pressures in the vessels can also be measured with the catheters.

Usually, a patient is given a premedication to reduce anxiety before undergoing one of these tests. The patient lies on a table under an x-ray camera. Often he will be able to view the picture that is being produced on a black-and-white TV monitor overhead. These tests are done with local anesthesia (usually Xylocaine) at the site where the blood vessel is entered. A small cut (about one-fourth inch) is made through the skin where the catheter is to be put into the vessel.

The most common risk is bleeding at the site of entering the vessel, though other complications like perforation of a vessel rarely occur. Question the doctor about the risks related to your specific test. As in the discussion of x-rays with dye or "contrast," a flushed or hot feeling may occur in these tests when dye is injected. Also, the body will try to eliminate the very dense dye quickly, and there is a tendency to become dehydrated, as urination considerably increases after a dye injection.

OTHER DYE STUDIES

Dye is placed into a variety of body spaces to better delineate them—the spinal canal (myelogram), the bronchial tree (bronchogram), abnormal communications between one organ and another (sinogram). Each of these tests has its own risks and potential to better delineate a problem. You must carefully question your physician to assess the risk-benefit trade-off of each test suggested for you. The questions later in this chapter are designed to help you do that.

This brief general overview covers only broad categories of commonly performed tests. Many other procedures exist to evaluate specific conditions and specific organs.

INFORMED CONSENT

Much has been written about informed consent. Any procedure or test that may have a significant complication associated with it requires informed consent. This means that you must sign a paper stating the doctor (or person who understands the procedure well, depending on the law and/or policy where you live) has explained to you in nontechnical terms the test that is proposed and the risk of all complications, including death even if that is a one-in-a-million chance. To give informed consent, you have to be mentally competent and not under the influence of mind-altering or sedating drugs or preoperative medications at the time the test and its risks are explained to you. The fact that the test and complications have been explained to you is usually witnessed by a second person not involved in (but who understands) the performing of the test. You, the witness, and the person informing you will all be required to sign a paper stating that the test, its risks, and potential complications have been explained to you and that you understand them. If anesthesia is required, the risks of anesthesia must also be explained, and this is included in the informed consent. If any pieces of organs (biopsies) or organs are to be removed, you may also be asked to permit these to be used to teach physicians in training about the disease process these organs demonstrate.

The real difficulty in informed consent is deciding what constitutes significant side effects or complications. Obviously, if informed consent were signed for every blood test and x-ray done, literally millions of consent forms would have to be signed every day; thus, "significant" is generally interpreted to mean complications that might result in increased need for medical care or longer hospitalization for the patient or any permanent disability. From the questions I have listed in the following section, you should be able to determine whether informed consent is in order for any procedure suggested for you. If it seems to be, but has not been mentioned, ask about it, and most important, if you are required to sign an informed consent, make sure you understand what the test involves and all risks before signing. If you don't, ask for simplification and clarification until you do.

Regardless of whether informed consent is required, however, you have the right and the obligation to know what studies you are going to be subjected to, why, and the potential risks, even if small.

The following list of questions will help you understand the role of medical tests in the evaluation or work-up of your symptoms, as well as what the tests themselves involve. As with most stresses in life, tests are not nearly as frightening if you know in advance what is going to happen.

THE PROCEDURES AS THEY RELATE TO YOUR SYMPTOMS

♦ 1   **How will this test aid in the diagnosis or therapy of my illness?**

As mentioned at the beginning of this chapter, tests are done for a variety of reasons. The doctor always has a mental scheme of how the work-up should or will be conducted, but because he is so familiar with this sort of work-up or is a poor communicator, he may inadvertently neglect to outline things in detail to you. If this happens, start asking questions.

◆ 2   Will I need to be hospitalized?

For some tests you do need to be hospitalized and this may entail additional arrangements for you. Ask if you have an alternative—can it be done as either an inpatient or an outpatient—and decide which is best for your needs, as well as your insurance coverage.

◆ 3   Will other tests need to be done?

Sometimes if one test is "positive" or "negative," that is the extent of the necessary procedures. At other times, a test's or procedure's results may indicate that others need to be performed, *or* from the beginning several tests may be planned to better delineate a problem. Examples: If your symptoms suggest bladder infection, probably the only test done will be a urine culture. If you have fevers, chills, loss of weight, and no abnormal physical findings, several blood, urine, and x-ray tests may be ordered simultaneously.

◆ 4   Will I need other tests in the future, or will I need this test repeated?

This offers further clarification of 3. If tests are being used to follow therapy or to follow a benign condition which could become life-threatening or debilitating, the same test may be repeated several times. Generally, the same chance of side effects exists from one time to the next, but your familiarity with the test will make it easier for you.

◆ 5   Are there simpler or less risky ways to evaluate my symptoms?

There are always many ways to approach the work-up of a patient's symptoms; the same is true of following therapy. No two physicians will proceed in exactly the same way. If you indicate to your doctor that you are interested in discussing alternative approaches, he can discuss this with you, as well as the risk-benefit information (of course, if you feel comfortable with the approach suggested, this question need not be presented). Remember, the less risk involved often means a smaller chance of diagnosis and more tests ultimately (but not always).

If you are a 45-year-old smoker whose x-ray has revealed a small nodule near the edge of your lung, a nodule that was not there one year ago, and you are otherwise healthy, I might suggest starting with a percutaneous aspiration of the nodule through a needle. Even though I know you have a significant risk of lung collapse, I recommend this because the diagnostic yield is quite high. Another physician may suggest a bronchoscopy first (see earlier in this chapter), which has less risk of lung collapse but lower yield. You have a significant chance of having to go on to a needle aspiration in the future if the bronchoscopy yield is negative. Also, he will have spent more money and lost some time in making the diagnosis by recommending a safer procedure.

Other factors also enter into a suggested work-up, including the skill of those performing certain tests and the availability of tests at the institution where you are being evaluated.

♦ 6. **What if no diagnosis is made?**

It may be that even though the appropriate test or series of tests is done, a diagnosis cannot be made. Depending on how serious the symptoms sound to the physician— e.g., if similar symptoms are not usually associated with serious or life-threatening diseases—he may elect to observe you and see if the symptoms go away. However, if the symptoms seem ominous, he may obtain consultation from another doctor, redo some tests, or even go as far as exploratory surgery to make a diagnosis.

♦ 7. **Do I have any particular risk factors for any of the tests?**

Risks of procedures will be addressed in the next section; but sometimes, features peculiar to a particular patient will increase the risk from a particular test. For example, patients with a certain type of kidney disease may be at risk of worsening kidney function if they undergo kidney x-rays with dye injections (IVP). This may be an irreversible and, therefore, unacceptable risk. Percutaneous needle aspirations of lung nodules are more risky because of increased risk of lung collapse in patients with emphysema.

♦ 8.   Will my insurance cover the costs of tests done either inside or outside of the hospital?

Clarify in advance the amount of the tests' costs that insurance will cover. Be certain about stipulations covering only inpatient or only outpatient tests. Most procedures are quite expensive, and if not covered by insurance, your doctor or hospital may be able to make some special arrangements for you.

THE TEST OR PROCEDURE

♦ 1.   Please explain to me exactly what you are going to do during this test before you start.

The greatest fear you will have before a test is that you don't know what is going to happen. This fear can be greatly reduced if the person doing the test takes time to go over it step by step before starting.

♦ 2   How long will it take?

Obviously, if you have come for a test expecting it to take fifteen minutes, and you find it taking three hours, your plans for the day are going to be disrupted *and* you are going to start thinking something is going wrong with the test. To avoid this, make sure you know in advance about how long it will take.

♦ 3   Can I expect any unusual feelings, pain, or sensations?

Again, this is to help you be better prepared for the tests and to avoid becoming frightened because something occurs which you did not expect. For example, if your throat is being numbed for a bronchoscopy or gastroscopy, you may start to feel as if you can't breathe or swallow. If you know about this sensation ahead of time, that this is simply an effect of anesthesia, you will not panic. Also, if you know about the hot sensations of dye injections, they will be easier to handle.

♦ 4 **What are the risks of this test, and how often do they happen? Am I at particular risk?**

Especially if you are having several tests, ask about the risks of each individually. Find out if you will be required to sign an informed consent for any of them. Most important, before you undertake a procedure, be sure that the potential risk of complications is acceptable, because you can't change your mind afterward. Also, ask whether any aspects of your personal situation—e.g., age, other illness, medications—will increase your risk.

♦ 5. **Are there special instructions to follow before or after this test?**

Many tests are preceded by special preparation. This may vary from several days of special diet, to enemas, to just not eating for a few hours before the test. Failure to follow pre- or post-test instructions may make it necessary to repeat the test and increase your costs, and it may increase the likelihood of complications. Also, you may be instructed not to drive or do work that requires clear thinking after the test because of premedications. Often you will be instructed not to drive for several hours.

♦ 6 **Will I need to be seen after the test is done?**

Make sure you have a follow-up appointment (if necessary to check for possible complications), especially to get results of tests that have been completed. Often so many tests are being done on patients, it is easy to overlook one. However, if an appointment is made to review test results, this won't happen. Some other arrangement that is mutually acceptable for passing on this information can be made if it fits the situation better, e.g., a telephone call or relaying results to the patient's primary doctor who will give them to the patient.

♦ 7 How will I know if a complication is occurring?

While it may seem obvious that one would recognize a complication of a procedure, this is not necessarily true. Complications may begin subtly. A bit of lightheadedness when you stand up, a slight sensation of breathlessness, a slight fever; sometimes these are important warning signs, sometimes not.

♦ 8 What should I do if I experience a complication?

Most complications are very mild and can be handled by careful observation at home. Others are potentially life-threatening and must be looked for immediately. This will vary from procedure to procedure, and will have to be clarified for each test.

♦ 9 Are there any side effects I should not be concerned about?

As important as it is to know signs of serious complications, it is just as important to know about minor side effects of the procedure and premedication that can be expected to occur and should not be of particular concern. It is also important to know if there are special ways to deal with these side effects.

   With answers to these questions and some general knowledge of tests you will undergo, your fears should be considerably lessened.

CHAPTER SIX

◆

GETTING
A SECOND
OPINION:
WHEN AND
WHAT
TO ASK

◆

Getting a "second opinion" is a much talked about approach to medical care in these days of the educated consumer and the astronomic costs of health care delivery.

A second opinion refers to the patient's seeing two separate physicians for recommendations regarding the same set of symptoms. What this generally means is the patient's asking a second doctor or other qualified professional about a particular proposed treatment, diagnosis, or other aspect of an illness.

A second opinion can be initiated by the patient or his physician, but is usually suggested by the patient. It may involve obtaining the services of a specialist in the disease process involved, or it may mean asking another physician in the same field, e.g., another gynecologist regarding a proposed hysterectomy, how he would approach the problem.

A few points need to be clarified before going into the details of obtaining a second opinion.

Often the second opinion will vary slightly, if at all, from your physician's assessment. However, if it does, you should remember that medicine is not an exact science. It is mostly an art, and issues are rarely black and white. What works for one person may be inappropriate for another. For example, your doctor may recommend a particular approach to therapy for you that is different from the approach he is recommending for the same illness in your neighbor. This is because the disease in you may really be different from the disease in your neighbor, or you may have other individual characteristics, e.g., age or sex, or other problems which dictate a different approach. While certain approaches to a given problem or illness are widely accepted among doctors, the specific methods of achieving a certain treatment or result vary widely— both from one institution to another and from one doctor to another. This does not mean one is right and one is wrong; it simply might (and usually does) mean there are many ways to reach the same goal. Therefore, a second opinion is just that, an opinion. How to evaluate the second opinion, I will discuss later in this chapter.

Questions of right and wrong are usually not the

main issue in obtaining a second opinion. Usually, the question boils down to whether one approach may be more acceptable than another. For example, you may have had a "gallbladder attack" and have been told you need surgery for gallstones, but you are deathly afraid of surgery and you wish an alternative, if one exists. You find out there is a process by which gallstones can be dissolved—albeit with some side effects—but you prefer this approach and ask to see a physician who does this type of therapy. One approach is not right and the other wrong; one is simply more acceptable to the patient under these circumstances.

Second, it is usually not offensive to one's primary physician to suggest that you wish a second opinion. Most physicians realize that when patients receive a very serious diagnosis, like cancer, or a recommended treatment that is risky, like some surgeries, they will be frightened and may want confirmation of the situation. The physician himself may recommend a second opinion. What is important in this tumultuous time in a patient's life is that a previously good relationship with the primary physician not be disturbed or destroyed because of a breakdown in communication. It is, for example, much more preferable for you to discuss your desire for a second opinion with your doctor—and, of course, it is his obligation to make you feel at ease in so doing—than for him to receive unannounced a report from a fellow doctor who has obviously been seeing you for the same problem. Always keep in mind that, from both yours and your doctor's point of view, communication, in this, as in any interpersonal relationship, is the key to maintaining the relationship. While a patient may at times feel uneasy about a treatment plan or its risks or about a diagnosis, it is often difficult for one to know when one should initiate a discussion about obtaining a second opinion. Following are some guidelines for you in making this decision.

♦ **1.   Is the diagnosis uncertain?**

Nothing is going to make you feel more uncomfortable than having an undiagnosed set of symptoms. If a number of tests have been completed without definitive results, you aren't going to feel any better that there are a bunch of negative results in your chart.

Often at this stage of a work-up, the physician also feels quite frustrated and is open to obtaining consultation—and may even suggest it. Certainly another doctor might think of something the family doctor hasn't, or he might have seen a similar case presentation that will help in making the diagnosis.

♦ 2.   Is the diagnosis life-threatening?

Risk of dying certainly is a legitimate reason for a patient to seek a second opinion. To receive a diagnosis like cancer often leaves the patient's life suddenly in a shambles. However, of all the possible reasons proposed for getting a second opinion, this is the least likely to vary from one physician to another. A diagnosis like cancer is based almost always on the study by pathologists of actual pieces of tissue that show cancer cells; it is rarely, if ever, based only on the patient's symptoms. Therefore, it may well allow you to face the situation better to hear a life-threatening diagnosis from two separate doctors, but this type of diagnosis is unlikely to change. The approach to therapy may, however, be quite different, and this will be discussed later.

♦ 3   Is the therapy controversial, experimental, or risky?

Often the diagnosis is not really in question, but rather it is the suggested therapy that is causing problems. Since a number of types of therapy may be available for a certain illness, you may well wish to ask another doctor what his approach would be in your particular case. This should be done, though, only if you feel the therapy is particularly difficult to handle, has a high risk of unacceptable side effects, is experimental, or has only a small chance of success, and if you feel uneasy about it and have informed your own physician about your concerns. Remember that your neighbor with the same illness may be receiving a completely different therapy because of his unique problems or if the expression of the disease in him is quite different from yours.

♦ **4 Is the therapy not working?**

If the therapy you are on does not seem to be effective in controlling the disease, the first step should be to ask your doctor about alternative drugs or other approaches. However, if he is unaware of other approaches or unwilling to change his approach, it is legitimate to see another doctor, possibly in this case one who specializes in your type of illness.

♦ **5 Are tests or procedures that entail considerable risk, e.g., permanent disability or death, being suggested?**

It is literally impossible for a person not thoroughly versed in medicine to be able to sort out whether or not he needs the load of tests and other procedures often suggested in the work-up of a disease. To be more informed, read Chapter 5 on what you need to know about a specific procedure. If you feel that a procedure has been proposed that has an unacceptable risk of side effects or death no matter what its potential yield, you should seek a different point of view. Sometimes, it is necessary to undergo a procedure even though it is risky because of the potential benefit, but it is important to hear that from two separate sources.

♦ **6 Do you want another approach?**

Certainly, philosophies of how to handle illnesses vary as much as political party affiliation. Some doctors are very aggressive in pursuing a particular diagnosis and in treatment even though the patient might be old and frail and the disease is not life-threatening. Others adopt a conservative, minimal-procedure, lower-cost, wait-and-see approach. Either might be appropriate depending on the situation. For example, an 80-year-old man with heart disease may have a spot on his x-ray that suggests a cancer. Because of other illness and general expected survival, one physician may elect not to undertake a diagnostic work-up. He feels that the discomfort and information gained will not significantly alter the man's therapy or prognosis and will cause him some discomfort. A second feels it is important to document the diagnosis and undertake some therapy because the role of the illness in the man's future is uncertain. In the process, the patient will have to undergo tests that will entail some risk and discomfort but the doctor feels the benefit is greater.

Other differences in approach to medical care may be at issue. One of these may be control. Some patients want more control over their care than doctors are willing to give, and vice versa. A second opinion may help clarify the amount of control the patient should have, or is able to manage. Can the patient, for example, adjust his own steroids or insulin in appropriate situations, or would allowing him to do this endanger his life?

◆ 7   **Is the doctor competent?**

All doctors must go through a licensing procedure to be allowed to practice medicine. Even so, some doctors are clearly not well versed in the areas they are supposed to be treating. Other times the doctor may be quite competent in the area of your illness, but he has not been able to communicate this to you. In either case, your confidence in him may have faltered and a second opinion is useful, even if it only reaffirms your faith in your own doctor.

◆ 8   **Does the physician want it?**

Most doctors have the best interest of their patients foremost in their mind and readily recognize areas in which their knowledge is deficient. Thus, it is not uncommon for the physician to suggest that you see another doctor for a second opinion. Also, a good doctor will recognize when a patient is feeling uncertain, frightened or insecure about something and may suggest that for the patient's peace of mind, a second opinion be obtained.

HOW TO MAINTAIN THE RELATIONSHIP WITH YOUR FAMILY DOCTOR

Obtaining a second opinion should not be a secretive act that results in bad feelings and antagonizes your family doctor or jeopardizes your relationship with him. Of course, if he is the one suggesting the second opinion, there is no problem. If, however, the initiating comes from you, the best approach is to be open and upfront from the beginning. If you handle the situation well, you will almost never encounter resistance from your doctor, and in fact, he will probably be supportive. You should tell him in advance that you intend to seek a second opinion and should do it, as you would in any relationship, in as diplomatic a manner as possible.

It is important to discuss this with your physician in advance so that he doesn't feel undermined or surprised when he receives a report about you from another doctor. I would suggest something like the following approach:

"You know, Dr. ....., you've been my doctor for five years, and I have gained a lot of confidence in you, but I am a little scared of the side effects of this new drug. Before I try it, I would like to be sure there is not something safer. Do you think we could ask one of those heart specialists if there is something else?"

Or:
"Dr. ....., I have the greatest respect for you and I appreciate your frankness and honesty, but I can't quite cope with a mastectomy yet. I think I need to hear the diagnosis from someone else before I can make a decision like that about my body."

The doctor, from his point of view, should be gracious and accepting of the patient's decision, especially in trying circumstances, and make it as easy and as comfortable as possible for her to obtain a second opinion. In this setting, it should not be difficult to maintain the primary care doctor/patient rapport.

WHERE TO GO FOR A SECOND OPINION AND HOW TO GO ABOUT IT

The difficult part of getting a second opinion is in finding a doctor from whom to get it. If seeking the second opinion is the doctor's suggestion, you may wish to ask him to recommend two other physicians and pick one to see. Your doctor, however, is likely to suggest other physicians who have a philosophy similar to his because, generally, these would be the colleagues to whom he is closest and for whom he has a good deal of respect.

Other ways of finding doctors are to call your local hospital or local branch of the medical society and ask for the names of two qualified physicians who practice medicine of the type that includes your problem. A more "hit-or-miss" approach (because you have less assurance of the doctor's reputation) is to use the Yellow Pages. I would not encourage this means of choosing a physician unless no other option is feasible.

Occasionally, especially in small towns, finding a second qualified physician may be difficult, and you may have to go to a nearby larger medical center. Often the second opinion in such instances is welcomed by your doctor.

Again, remember, don't do this behind your doctor's back (see preceding discussion). Ask your doctor for a summary of your records to be sent to the other doctor or to take along when you go. You should call and make an appointment, although your doctor may agree to do this once you have selected another physician.

Most doctors will readily see you for this purpose and will wish to send a report back to your doctor.

Two points should be emphasized: First, the second doctor will likely redo much of the work-up that has already been done by your physician. In addition to the history and physical exam, this might also include some tests or procedures. Ask if any of the results already available might suffice in order to reduce the number of studies.

Second, inquire about the cost of the doctor's evaluation and check in advance whether your insurance covers this. If the cost is prohibitive for you, ask if a reduced charge or payment plan can be arranged.

If the second opinion differs from your doctor's, ask both physicians why they have taken the one point of view and not the other. Ultimately, however, you will have to make a decision. Occasionally, a third opinion is warranted, but be careful not to get into the dilemma of "doctor-hopping" and never making a decision.

◆

UNDERSTANDING
THE ROLE OF
THE SPECIALIST
CONSULTANT

◆

At times during the course of your illness, unusual problems may arise for which you will require the services of a specialist in consultation.

What is a specialist consultation? A specialist is a doctor who is particularly knowledgeable in a limited area of medicine. He may be a *sub*specialist in a field of internal medicine: for example, a gastroenterologist is particularly knowledgeable about the gut and other abdominal organs; a cardiologist is particularly knowledgeable about the heart. On the other hand, the specialist may be from a completely different field of medicine. He may specialize in ophthalmology (eyes), obstetrics-gynecology (female medicine), or orthopedics (bones and joints). Reasons one might need or benefit from consultation with a specialist will be explored here.

First, you must understand the role of the specialist in your care. The most important thing to remember when you visit a specialist is that he is a consultant. He will talk to you, examine you and make suggestions or recommendations regarding your diagnosis or care, or he will perform a predetermined surgical or other procedure. While you necessarily will have a relationship with the specialist, your primary relationship will continue with your primary doctor. The specialist will send a written evaluation of your visit with recommendations to your doctor.

Remember that your primary doctor knows you much better than the specialist because he has cared for you over time. (For example, your primary doctor knows whether you follow instructions well, whether your family relationships influence how you cope with your illness, whether you are prone to drug reactions.) This is where the art of medicine interacts with the science. Your doctor will review the recommendations of the specialist, and carry out those which are likely to be in your best interest and improve your well-being. He may modify or omit some suggestions because he knows you well enough to know they would not work for you.

For example, you are a busy model. The specialist recommends that you change your medication to four times a day instead of your usual twice a day. Your internist knows you occasionally miss doses on your current schedule, and he, in fact, changed you to twice a day so you could be more compliant. He decides to leave you on your current twice a day schedule but to add another drug which the specialist recommended be taken just after the first drug, also twice a day. He reasons that since you are taking drugs anyway, you are likely to take both drugs twice a day.

You may need periodic reassessment by the specialist, and your internist will be the best person to arrange this follow-up.

Now let us look at some of the reasons you might need to see a specialist for consultation.

◆ 1   You have an unusual disease or unusual manifestation of a common disease

A general internist will be familiar with, and his knowledge current in, common illnesses. However, he may or may not have a thorough knowledge of an unusual illness and may wish to ask for recommendations from someone who is likely to know the most current information about that disease and probably treats more such cases. For example, an internist will often feel comfortable treating asthma. However, he may wish to involve a subspecialist, a pulmonary (lung) internist, in the care if the patient develops a complication of asthma called allergic bronchopulmonary aspergillosis. Or your internist may wish consultation from a pulmonary physician if you develop the rare illness alveolar proteinosis, which he probably has not previously treated.

◆ 2   You have an unusually fast progression or severe symptoms of your disease.

Occasionally, an illness follows a very rapid or severe downhill course. This can be extremely frustrating for the physician, the patient, and the family. Under these circumstances, a consultation by an expert may occasionally uncover some factor in the illness which can reverse or stem the progression, or some medication which has been overlooked. For example, a relatively well-controlled asthma patient has had a marked increase in symptoms and hospitalizations over the last year. A careful history reveals that about one year ago she began taking Inderal for high blood pressure, and this is a well-known cause of asthma attacks in susceptible patients. Usually, however, this type of thing does not happen, and the value of the consultation lies in the assurance it gives the referring doctor and the patient/family that everything possible is being done.

◆ **3   You have failed to respond to therapy**

Failure to get adequate relief from symptoms can also be a big source of frustration to both you and your physician. This is a frequent impetus to seek a consultation. Since the specialist sees many patients with your illness, he may know very recent developments in therapy or special techniques with known therapy which may improve your response. Again, if neither the specialist nor your internist is able to give you complete relief, you will at least have the assurance all avenues have been explored. In situations such as this, periodic reassessments by a specialist may be important, in that new developments in many areas of internal medicine occur literally every day.

◆ **4   You develop a new problem or complication of your illness requiring a different type of medical expertise**

Most types of chronic illness follow a course of many years. Sometimes the disease or the therapy affects other organs of the body or causes progressive deterioration of the original target organ. These changes may require the expertise of a variety of doctors.

Consider diabetes mellitus, an extremely common illness in North America. A number of diabetics will, after 15 or 20 years, develop problems with their eyes which may vary from cataracts to bleeding at the back of the eye. Many of the eye problems require the technical expertise of an ophthalmologist. Some diabetics may develop severe nerve deficits requiring the services of a neurologist and vessel changes that require bypass grafts performed by vascular surgeons.

A patient with rheumatoid arthritis may have progressive destruction of joints and bone tissue which would make the hands useless and the sufferer unable to walk were it not for the corrective surgery and the artificial joints that an orthopedist can offer.

Thus, in many ways, many chronic illnesses have both medical and surgical aspects, and their successful treatment depends on a close relationship between your primary internist and his colleagues.

♦ 5   You require a special procedure or test

Often a primary doctor or general internist will be able to treat an illness, but he may lack the special training to carry out a particular test or procedure that you require. If you have a duodenal ulcer, you may need an endoscopy, in which your esophagus, stomach, and upper small intestine are looked at through a finger-sized, flexible, black tube carrying fiberoptic light bundles (called a gastroscope or endoscope). Generally, only persons who specialize in "gut" medicine (gastroenterologists) or some surgeons would have the training to do this procedure, and your internist may ask for a consultation specifically for the procedure to be done.

♦ 6.   You or your physician wishes a second opinion

The circumstances under which you or your doctor wish to get a second opinion can be quite variable (see Chapter 6 on getting a second opinion). Often a second opinion is obtained from another doctor with similar training, but there are many times when asking a specialist for a second opinion is appropriate. In this type of case, there is an overlap between consultations and second opinions. If you have been told by a lung specialist that you have inoperable (or incurable) lung cancer, for which there is no good treatment, you may wish to get a consultation from a cancer doctor (oncologist) or a thoracic surgeon. The points of view may vary and if they do give you conflicting opinions, remember that this is probably because no single approach is "right" and several alternative approaches may be equally sound. You must choose the best for you.

WHO SHOULD ASK FOR THE CONSULTATION?

The correct answer is either you or your doctor. Most often your physician will perceive the need for specialist help or know when to ask for help before you recognize a need for it; most physicians recognize their limitations so that they initiate calls for consultation when they feel they need the benefit of a physician with broader or different expertise, training, or knowledge. Your doctor will know a group of specialists in a variety of fields to whom he has sent other patients, and whom he has found to be helpful, reliable, and professional.

Your internist or his staff, when it has been decided to request consultation, should either make arrangements for the consultation or instruct you how to do so. Then he will provide to the specialist a summary of your problems and relevant medication and test data, along with specific questions for which he is requesting help in managing your case. This will allow the specialist to focus on those areas and provide your doctor with the most meaningful data. After he sees you, the specialist will send a written report of the visit along with recommendations to your internist.

If you feel that you have problems that fit into any of the above-suggested categories for getting specialist consultation but your doctor has not asked for it, discuss the possibility with him. This should be your first step, rather than going directly to a specialist, because it is important to preserve your relationship with your primary doctor. In fact, he may be surprised to find you have concerns about which he was not aware. Or you might have read about a "new" approach he hasn't heard about or has little knowledge of, and he may well view your request as a learning experience for himself. You may find he hasn't asked for consultation because he didn't think you would want it. In any case, most often he will agree to ask for consultation, if you are concerned.

If in the occasional circumstance you find your internist is averse to your request and you do not feel he has a good reason for his opinion, or he seems disinterested in your concerns, you can initiate specialist consultation on your own. However, if this degree of disruption occurs in your relationship with your primary doctor, it may be time to change to someone with whom you can work more easily.

If arrangements are being made for you to see a specialist, for whatever reason, you should have two sets of questions clearly in mind. First, make sure you have the facts about the consultation from your doctor, and second, make sure you know what you want to learn from the consultant. Following are questions that cover both situations.

QUESTIONS THAT SHOULD BE CLARIFIED WITH YOUR PRIMARY DOCTOR BEFORE YOU VISIT THE CONSULTANT

♦ 1 **Why are you sending me to a specialist?**

While you may have asked to be sent to a specialist, it more likely has been the request of your internist. If you have not discussed why he feels you need to see a specialist, you need to clarify the reason for your own information as well as to make sure this question is clearly addressed when you see the specialist.

♦ 2 **How much will consultation cost and will my insurance cover it?**

The cost of medical care being what it is, this may not be a minor concern. The cost of a consultation certainly is going to far exceed the cost of your regular office visit. If the reason for the consultation is unclear or a relatively minor problem to you, you may decide to wait a while before going *or* not to go. When cost is a factor, this should be discussed with your primary doctor. Also find out if your insurance will cover the expense.

♦ 3 **What if I decide against consultation?**

If for some reason (e.g., financial, difficulties in transportation) you decide not to see the specialist, it is important to discuss this with your doctor. This will allow him to rethink his management of your problem. As a second best approach, he may call a specialist and discuss your problems on the phone. Or he may negotiate with you to continue as is for the present, with the provision you see a specialist at a specified future time, if the worrisome problems continue. Or he may feel the consultation is critical to your care now, and may not feel comfortable caring for you without it. Whatever the case, it should be clear to both of you.

♦ **4   If the specialist suggests changes in medications, hospitalization, etc., should I do this or see you first?**

Different doctors have different relationships with the consultants they use. In some cases, your doctor may have such a well-established relationship with and such confidence in the consultant, he will ask you to follow recommendations before he has a chance to see you again. In other cases, if, say, surgery or other hospitalization is involved, or your doctor is not very familiar with the consultant, he may wish to review any recommendations before you implement them.

♦ **5   Will you want the specialist to follow me?**

If new or experimental drugs are going to be used or if you have surgery or other tests, the specialist may need to have follow-up appointments with you. Often if you have an advanced or hard-to-treat illness, the specialist may want to monitor your progress at, say, three-month intervals. Generally, this is perfectly okay with your internist, but again the critical element is that communication takes place so everyone involved knows what's going on. Also, it is usually best to arrange the follow-up through your primary doctor.

♦ **6   When should I see you after the consultation?**

Always be sure you have made arrangements for your own internist—who takes care of all your problems—

to see you after the consultation. Sometimes, so much scheduling and planning are going on, you forget to do this and proposed changes, tests, etc., can be neglected for months. Arranging follow-up will remind you and the doctor to check test results or review proposed medication changes or whatever the consultant has suggested.

♦ **7   If I need to be hospitalized for surgery or other reasons, will you see me in the hospital?**

It is important to arrange for your own doctor to be involved in your care in any hospitalization that may be required. If, for example, you are going to require gallbladder surgery and you are an insulin-dependent diabetic, your internist will be the best person to follow your blood sugar and insulin requirements during and after the surgery. Not only will he, because of his experience, expertise, and greater knowledge of your disease, be able to manage your medical problems, he will also know your peculiarities *and* it will be nice for you to see a familiar face.

QUESTIONS FOR YOUR CONSULTANT

What questions then should the *specialist* be able to answer for you? Well, you should know the specific reason for the consultation and make sure that reason is clear to the specialist and has been addressed by him before you leave the office. The burden in this respect falls on you because you, and not your primary doctor, are present at the consultation.

The exact questions you need to ask depend on the reason for the consultation. If, for example, the reason for the consultation is that you have failed to respond to therapy, you should have answers to this type of question before you leave:

1. ♦ Can you find any reasons why the treatment has not worked?
2. ♦ Can I make any changes in the way I take the medicine that will increase the effect of the drugs?

3. ♦ Are there other or newer treatments that can be
   tried?

If the reason for the consultation is that you have a
rare disease or unusual manifestation of a common
disease, you will want to know answers to these questions:

1. ♦ What is the cause of this illness?
2. ♦ What is the current therapy for this disease?
3. ♦ What is the prognosis?
4. ♦ If the disease progresses, are any new radical approaches (like organ transplant) feasible?
5. ♦ Is this illness hereditary?

From the general questions in Chapters 2 and 3 you
should be able to set out and *write down* before your
consultation a group of questions that will give you
the information you need from the consultant. Before
you leave make sure you find out if you will need any
special tests that the consultant has to schedule and
whether you will require any follow-up appointments
with him.

If during the consultation you feel some confusion
about the reason for the consultation or the kind of
information you seem to be getting from the consultant, it is possible the referring doctor's letter has not
arrived or his request may not have been clear to the
consultant. If you think this may be happening, it is a
good idea to say this diplomatically to the doctor and
suggest he give your doctor (called the "referring doctor"), a quick telephone call to clarify matters. You
might say something like, "I'm sorry, Dr. Jones, but I
don't remember Dr. Lee mentioning eye surgery,
since we hadn't tried all the medicines. Would you
mind giving him a call and see if that's what he had in
mind?"

CHAPTER EIGHT

◆

WHEN TO
CONSIDER
CHANGING
DOCTORS

◆

The relationship between doctor and patient is in many ways special and unlike the relationship one is likely to have with any other professional. It has a unique sort of intimacy. The doctor has an intimate knowledge of the patient's dearest possession—his health—and is entrusted with maintaining that as best he can. He often also has an intimate knowledge of family interactions and secrets, especially if he has cared for the family for years. Because of this, maintaining communication in the relationship is critical, and most doctor-patient relationships that are dissolved occur in the face of communication breakdown.

The termination of doctor-patient relationships is often not unlike divorces, possibly with strong feelings on both sides. Because it takes time and work to build a good doctor-patient rapport, and time for a doctor to really know and understand a patient's problems so that he can tailor care to that patient's specific needs, moving around from one doctor to another is usually not in your best interest. The doctor and the patient both have a considerable investment in any relationship that has been ongoing for some time, and care should be taken not to escalate simple annoyances or misunderstandings into major problems without discussion with the doctor. A simple explanation may solve what seemed to be a major crisis.

Many patients are not sure whether they should change doctors, but for some reason do not feel comfortable with their present situation. In the following pages, I will review what I think should be the elements of a good relationship and for what reasons one should (or should not) look for a new physician. Finally, I will suggest how you might break off a relationship and how you might go about looking for someone new.

When you are feeling a vague dissatisfaction with your doctor—as you might with anyone to whom you are close—ask yourself if the relationship has the following basic elements:

First, do you trust your physician? There are many areas in a doctor-patient relationship where trust is important. Does your physician act in your best interest even if monetary and other concerns are present? Does he maintain personal and family confidences?

Does he call for help in your care if his knowledge is inadequate to handle the situation? Is he honest with you about your health concerns? What are the things that are important to you in your relationship with your doctor, and do you trust his expertise in these areas?

Second, do you respect your doctor? Do you feel your doctor is competent in understanding and caring for your problem? Of course, doctors are closely regulated by the government and must take licensing examinations that recognize completion of studies, postgraduate training, and passing of exams establishing competence. In addition, most specialists in the various areas of medicine or surgery will have taken further sets of specialty examinations and will have certificates that acknowledge this.

Some patients also do not feel confident with a physician unless they feel comfortable with the way he conducts himself in his personal life and confident that he acts and dresses like a professional. Excessive drinking or other personal problems may erode your respect. Others might not care how a physician conducts his life outside the office. However you feel, you must be able to respect your doctor to trust him with your care.

Third, you must feel that the doctor understands your particular illness and family situation that results from that illness. If he does not want to take the time to get to know you, he is not going to develop an understanding of your problems and you are not likely to develop the mutual trust necessary to a good relationship.

Fourth, you must be able to communicate and feel comfortable discussing problems with the doctor in order to develop any of the previous three essentials of the relationship. If you are intimidated by the doctor, if he cuts you off in midsentence, if he patronizes you, or if he always seems in a hurry and you are not assertive, you may feel your problems are never fully discussed and resentments will build. On the other hand, remember communication is a two-way street. You *must* voice your concerns and questions—the doctor can't read your mind.

If you find that the essentials of a good relationship are present most of the time, there may still be some specific situations that occur and you are not sure what to do. Here are a few situations that occur commonly. The first group includes situations that I feel are usually *not* reasons to end a relationship:

1. A simple misunderstanding: A simple misunderstanding can easily be blown into a major crisis. An error in appointment times, failure to completely explain (or understand) how to take a medication, a disagreement over billing, etc., all fall into the category of misunderstanding and should be discussed *with* the doctor before it is magnified to something that can't be cleared up quickly. If you have established good communications in the past, this should not be difficult.

2. Human error: Doctors are human and occasionally errors are made. Errors rarely endanger the patient's health. These include most often inappropriate drug doses, use of incompatible or interacting drugs concurrently, failure to check on test results, forgetting to write a prescription, and similar things. Repeated errors are reason to be concerned; isolated instances that are rapidly corrected without harm to the patient should not be overemphasized.

3. Unrealistic expectations: We would all like to be cured of our ailments. Unfortunately, most illnesses that the internist treats can be controlled but not cured. It is easy to become discouraged when your disease progresses despite your doctor's best efforts. Sometimes such a situation calls for specialist consultation, a change in approach, or new tests. Many times, however, no matter what is done, the disease will continue to progress. It doesn't matter who the doctor is, he cannot cure the disease. Expecting him to will result in frustration for both of you.

4. "Friendly" advice: Talking to one's friend about mutual ailments often discloses that the approaches to treatment are different. This is *not* a reason to switch to the friend's doctor. The two illnesses may *not* be identical; other circumstances may be involved, e.g., concurrent illnesses or allergies. If the illnesses are identical, several approaches to therapy may be equally efficacious and the individual doctor probably

has good reasons to do what he does. If you have questions about your treatment after talking to someone with similar problems, make an appointment with your own doctor and ask about it.

5. Hearsay: Do not make hasty decisions based on rumors. Especially in small or close communities, it is easy for rumors to be started either about a physician's personal life or about professional conduct. You may hear rumors about a malpractice suit that has been brought. Remember that the initiation of a suit in no way establishes error on the part of the doctor, and rumors may be started with little factual basis. If you are disturbed by something you have heard, you can ask the doctor directly about the rumors you have heard.

The following is a list of situations in which you might seriously consider terminating a relationship:

1. An ethical/moral problem arises: Even in the best of relationships, a difference in personal philosophy can arise that will make it impossible for you and your doctor to work together. A usual situation might involve a patient with a terminal illness. The doctor might feel that he should try to maintain the patient's life as long as possible; the patient may not wish that any extraordinary efforts be used (like mechanical respirators), or the philosophies may be reversed. Either way the approaches to terminal illness are not compatible and may result in frustration and rancor when the patient gets to the stage where critical decisions need to be made.

2. Breakdown of communication: As in any relationship, the people involved can change to the extent that previously good communication no longer exists. Whether you feel you can no longer make yourself understood, are intimidated by the doctor, or whatever the reason, it is worthwhile trying to reestablish your rapport. Establishing new relationships is stressful and time-consuming, and sometimes the frustration you are feeling is due simply to a misunderstanding that can be easily cleared up. If not, however, it is best to find a new doctor.

3. Doctor too busy: As new doctors develop their practice, they become busier and busier. Most can tell when they are seeing the most patients possible but still are giving good care. A few, though, crowd many more patients into a day than they can care for effectively. If you are finding that you are getting less and less time per visit and having more difficulty getting appointments, you may wish to change to a less busy doctor.

4. Doctor unavailable or call coverage unavailable: Many medical problems occur after office hours. When this happens, you will call your doctor's answering service (or whatever prearrangement for nonoffice-hour problems you have), and speak to the doctor on call. If you repeatedly have difficulty reaching the covering physician or your physician during nonoffice hours, you may wish to change to someone who is more conscientious about availability. Of course, you must be careful not to make repeated "nuisance" calls that could easily wait until the next scheduled office hours for resolution.

5. Failure to follow through on new problems: New symptoms, medication side effects, or other problems often arise during the course of an illness. They should be reported promptly to your doctor in case action needs to be taken. When you are experiencing new problems, it may be impossible or difficult to remedy, or it may be something easily managed. In either case, you can expect the doctor to return your calls or arrange to see you and discuss the situation. If he repeatedly fails to return calls, become concerned. It is your responsibility, however, to report new problems; he may not be able to anticipate them.

6. You develop new problems requiring specialized care: Occasionally, you will develop problems requiring frequent care by a particular type of consultant. If you are soon going to require dialysis, for example, it may be more appropriate to be followed by a nephrologist (kidney specialist). Discuss this with your doctor.

7. Changing locations: Your doctor should be close to you. If you move, you may need to change physicians. Even if your physician is still reasonably located but the hospital he uses is too distant, you may wish to change.

8. Personality conflict: In any relationship, the possibility of a personality conflict exists. Usually, this is clear early in a relationship, but may develop later in response to a specific issue. Personality conflicts are very difficult to resolve, and terminating the relationship may be the only answer.

9. Conflicts involving fees: Sometimes disagreements over fees are easily resolved misunderstandings. Many times, however, fights about money can quickly poison a relationship. If you see this happening, and attempts at resolution have not been successful, it is better to end the relationship rather than become bitter.

Once you have identified a situation in which you feel sufficiently uncomfortable to wish to change doctors, how do you go about it?

Don't just leave without saying anything, though often this is the easiest thing to do. Arrange for an appointment for a consultation with your doctor. Explain your dissatisfaction. He may not even be aware of the situation that has caused your concern. Even if he is aware of the problem and a solution cannot be achieved, it is important that you tell him you will be seeing another doctor and, if possible, the doctor's name. This will alert him to expect a request from that physician to forward your records. You may be able to arrange for him to give you pertinent records which you can hand-carry to the new physician. In appropriate situations, e.g., if you will be requiring special care, if you are moving, etc., your doctor should be able to refer you to an appropriate physician. This kind of referral will likely enable you to get an early appointment with the new doctor.

If your relationship has so deteriorated that you do

not feel you can arrange a consultation, at least write the doctor a letter. He needs this feedback, so he may be made aware of your frustrations and hopefully take a good look at himself if he bears some responsibility for the breakdown of the relationship. Also, he should be told in the letter he will be receiving requests for your records and, if possible, from whom. You will probably have to sign a release allowing your records to be sent to the new doctor.

Severing the relationship is only half the battle. Now how do you go about finding a new doctor? If you have changed doctors because of moving or some similar reason, the answer is easy, as you can get a referral from your previous doctor. You may even be able to do this in less harmonious settings. However, often this is not the case, and unfortunately, there is no Better Business Bureau for doctors.

You can call the local chapter of the American or Canadian Medical Association and they will give you the names of several doctors of internal medicine in your area. Other sources of referral can be local hospitals or the telephone directory. The telephone directory is the least reliable of these, since the designations stating the physician's areas of specialization may simply reflect a particular interest of the doctor. It does not necessarily mean he has undergone a recognized program of training in that area. Doctors recommended by a local medical association or hospital will more reliably have completed such a program. In any case, you will probably want to arrange an interview session with two different doctors. If a doctor is unwilling to do this, he may be unwilling to sit down and discuss problems that arise as well. While you are meeting with the doctor, ask yourself: Can I talk easily with him about a variety of subjects? Does he seem concerned about *me*? Does he answer directly the questions I ask? Do we seem to have any personality conflicts?

IMPORTANT QUESTIONS TO ASK A NEW DOCTOR

♦ 1   Where do you hospitalize?

You should feel comfortable with the hospital your doctor uses and it should be reasonably accessible.

♦ 2   Do you have specialist certification?

To practice as an internist in the United States, a physician must pass a special examination given by the American Board of Internal Medicine. If he has passed this exam, he will have a certificate so stating.

In Canada, a similar examination is given by the Royal College of Physicians and Surgeons. Doctors who are successful on this exam, which includes both written tests and evaluation of patients, also receive certificates.

♦ 3   What are your provisions for office hours coverage?

Be sure you feel that coverage for emergency situations is adequate. It is too late once an emergency occurs to find out no one is available who knows your problems!

♦ 4   How long do you allow for appointments?

A doctor who allows ten minutes for a patient is unlikely to spend adequate time evaluating, explaining, and discussing problems with the patient. A first thorough exam usually takes a minimum thirty minutes and subsequent exams and discussions at least fifteen minutes.

♦ 5   What is your philosophy about care for terminally ill patients?

You probably are not terminally ill, nor should you expect to be in the near future. Nevertheless, you never know when this situation can occur, and it is wise to know your physician's basic philosophy in advance. Also, this is a question most physicians probably don't expect, and how the doctor handles it may give you an idea about how he handles difficult situations.

You may wish to ask other questions specifically relevant to your medical problems or that relate to the specific reasons you changed physicians, so that you do not get into another incompatible relationship.

If you have particular religious or other strong feelings about medical practices, e.g., blood transfusions, taking drugs, etc., you need also to find out the physician's willingness to work with you under these circumstances.

These questions will not guarantee a perfect match between you and the physician, but they will give you an impression about whether you can work with him. You undoubtedly will formulate more of your own as the interview goes on: If you do not feel comfortable asking questions that arise in your mind, this may not be the doctor for you.

◆

QUESTIONS
ABOUT
HOSPITALIZATION

◆

If your doctor tells you he wants you to go into the hospital for "some tests," let alone surgery, you are likely to suddenly feel a knot of anxiety (fear? panic?) in the pit of your stomach. Hardly anyone likes to be put in the hospital.

There are many reasons why people fear hospitalization. Hospitals are usually large, imposing structures, often somber in appearance. Once inside the lobby, you see people moving rapidly about, but you feel out of place. They are dressed in uniforms of one type or another and speak an English that seems more a foreign language because it is sprinkled with unfamiliar words and phrases. You stop to ask for information and feel stupid when your instruction-giver uses some of these foreign words and you have to ask for an interpretation. He stops, smiles sweetly but a bit patronizingly, then starts again slowly and in simple terms.

Aside from the ambiance of the hospital, most think of it as the other world. Going to the hospital means, doesn't it, that you are really sick, imperfect? We tend to think of our healthy selves as unblemished and somehow invulnerable. A trip to the hospital, benign as it may be, suddenly reminds us of our potential vulnerability, and that is very unsettling. The prospect of being sick, of being "invalid" and overwhelmed by an invisible enemy vaporizes our defenses and undermines our self-image. No wonder fear is our most common response to the symbol of illness in our society, the hospital.

For the elderly, the prospect of being hospitalized often symbolizes the end. They think of it as the place old folks go to die; they often aren't wrong.

Sometimes patients hate the hospital because they know it's a place where their bodies will be violated by needles, probed, mashed over and over, exposed to radiation, etc. Their privacy is nonexistent; and they are likely to eat drab, overdone food and never have a good night's sleep.

Whatever your reason, I'll bet you hate the idea of going to the hospital. The best way to handle your fears and assure yourself you aren't going to run into any unpleasant surprises is to ask plenty of questions ahead of time, and understand exactly what is going to take place, when and why. You don't know what to ask? Yes, you do. Read through the following questions and ask the ones that apply to you. I have divided them into four categories: (1) those pertaining to the hospital, (2) those regarding the tests themselves or changes in the therapy, (3) those relating to the means of payment, and (4) those regarding surgical procedures, if that is the reason for admission.

THE HOSPITAL

♦ **1   Where do I go when I reach the hospital, and what time should I arrive?**

Hospitals are big imposing buildings. If the doctor gives you instructions on how to get to the admissions area and when to get there, you will feel much more relaxed. After that, you pray for a friendly receptionist. Usually, hospitals will want you to arrive in the late morning, after discharges are made.

♦ **2   What should I take to the hospital? Are there any specific instructions?**

You are usually encouraged to bring very little to the hospital in the way of money or jewelry, because it can be easily stolen from your bedside table. Safe boxes are usually available to store goods if you for some reason do bring something of value. Most hospitals allow you to wear your own pajamas and robe; others do not, so you will have to ask. Also, some hospitals will not allow you to bring in things like TVs and radios.

♦ **3   Can I leave my car at the hospital?**

The hospital may or may not have facilities for this. It may depend on the security available for long-term parking as well as spaces available. Usually, it is best to have someone bring you to the hospital anyway, as you may not feel up to driving when you are discharged.

♦ **4   What ward or floor will I be admitted to?**

The more information you have in advance, the less strange the hospital will seem and the more relaxed you will feel. Also, you will be able to let your family know where you will be in advance.

♦ **5   What are the visiting hours? Are there restrictions on visitors?**

You can make yourself loved by the nursing staff by letting family and friends know in advance the rules for visiting hours, number of visitors allowed at a time, and whether or not children are allowed to come to the floor or to your room.

♦ **6   Do I have a choice of a private or semiprivate room, and will I have a telephone?**

Most modern hospitals have telephones in the rooms. Whether you will get a private or semiprivate room is often open to chance, unless you specifically ask for a private room and are willing to pay for it or your insurance will pay for it (most policies don't). Even so, if on the day of admission all private rooms are taken either for isolation of infected patients or for other reasons, you still may have to settle for a semiprivate. If you aren't satisfied, you may be able to get what you want in a day or so.

♦ **7   Does the hospital follow any special rules or have any special procedures I should be aware of?**

The preceding questions should cover most of your concerns, but occasionally a hospital has a particular set of rules, say, relating to the religious affiliation of the hospital. Knowing these in advance can avoid embarrassment later or prevent uncomfortable situations.

♦ **8   Is there a chaplain of my faith available or on call at the hospital?**

If you are religious and there is any possibility of something going wrong during the hospitalization, e.g., if you are being admitted for a major operation, you may wish to know of the availability of a chaplain and chapels. Some hospitals hold denominational or nondenominational services as well.

♦ 9 Does the hospital allow passes?

Many hospitals have systems whereby patients can leave the hospital for periods of hours to a couple of days. If you are admitted for diagnostic tests and little is done on weekends or evenings, you may wish to go out on pass.

ADMISSIONS FOR TESTS / PROCEDURES / CHANGES IN TREATMENT

♦ 1 Why are you recommending the tests (therapy) for which I am to be hospitalized?

Know what is going on with you: Does the internist feel you have some serious illness he is looking for? Or why is your present therapy failing? Further, you may find out that he is doing studies to see if you should have, e.g., open-heart surgery, which you are completely unwilling to have. That being the case, there would be no need to waste time and money doing preliminary studies.

♦ 2 Can these studies or therapy changes be done as an outpatient in my case?

A variety of reasons exist for choosing to do tests as an inpatient. The patient can be watched for complications; the patient requires sedation impairing judgment; a series of studies can be more efficiently handled as an inpatient; convenience to the patient; insurance covers more than when done as an outpatient. However, it may be that the main reason is that your doctor's patients tend to prefer inpatient evaluation.

He may have suggested this because he assumes you want it or it is his habit. You may be able to be managed as an outpatient, and this may be most convenient for you. It certainly is cheaper for you if you have no insurance coverage.

◆ **3   If I can make outpatient arrangements, will my insurance still cover cost?**

I repeat this as a special, critical question because tests are very expensive. Make sure all the insurance forms are filled out and submitted as soon as the tests are done. You will probably have to do the checking with your insurance company ahead of time to see if the tests would be covered as an outpatient.

◆ **4   How long am I likely to be hospitalized?**

You need this information to prepare for time off from your job, to arrange for baby-sitting, etc. However, hospital stays are unpredictable and it is wise to leave a leeway of at least a couple of days in case something unplanned comes up.

◆ **5   Will I be examined by anyone other than you after I am admitted?**

Many large hospitals are teaching hospitals and, as such, have residents or house staff who are postgraduate doctors gaining the experience needed to qualify in their particular field (e.g., internal medicine). Often one or more of these training physicians will admit and examine you and have some degree of responsibility for you in the hospital. You may also be seen by medical students. Besides the training physician, you may be seen by other specialists, depending upon what your problem entails.

◆ **6   If any of my tests are "positive" (abnormal), will that increase my hospital stay?**

Depending upon *why* you are having studies done, and what they are, the results of initial tests may suggest the need for further studies or treatment. This will increase your stay.

◆ **7   What are the risks of the studies (therapies) for which I am being hospitalized?**

You may decide, once you have heard the risks involved, that you don't want to go through with the tests. However, generally, the doctor will have recommended risky tests only if he thinks they are very important to your health evaluation. It is important you understand if this is the case, so that you can decide beforehand if you are willing to take the risks.

♦ 8   If I have complications, how much is my hospital stay likely to increase?

While this type of question does not have an exact answer because each patient is different, certain complications (or side effects) may be quite common and the increase in hospital time fairly predictable.

♦ 9   If complications or side effects occur, are there specialists available who can respond quickly?

If you were having a study of the bowel done called a colonoscopy, and the rare complication of tearing of the bowel occurred, you would like to know that surgeons and anesthesiologists were readily available to do the emergency surgery necessary. Some smaller hospitals do not have this type of coverage. If you are having studies with serious risks in a hospital that does not have on-site coverage like that, find out what the provisions to handle these complications are. Then decide whether you feel they are satisfactory.

FINANCIAL ARRANGEMENTS

♦ 1   Will my insurance cover the entire cost or, if not, how much?

Needless to say, hospital costs and tests can wipe out one's savings rapidly. Even having to pay 10 or 20 percent of a bill may be a burden. You will have to talk to your insurance company to find out exactly what is covered. Do this before you make any other plans for the hospitalization.

♦ 2   Will I need to put any money up as a deposit when I am admitted?

Even when insurance is likely to cover the costs, some hospitals require a cash deposit on admission. If this is difficult for you to do, occasionally it will be waived.

♦ 3   **What kind of arrangements for payment can be made?**

You may have to discuss this with the hospital rather than the doctor. You should call their accounting department prior to your stay and find out their policy. If you have to pay even 10 to 20 percent of the bill, this may be a sizable amount, and you may have to spread it over several months. Also, many hospitals will write off a percentage of the bill if you are unable to pay.

ADMISSIONS FOR SURGERY

♦ 1   **Why are you recommending this surgery for me now?**

Be clear why your doctor feels this surgery is indicated *now.* This should not be a "challenging" or "adversarial" question. It is an attempt to clearly understand your medical problems and why this operation would be wise at this time.

♦ 2   **How long before the surgery do I need to be admitted?**

Many times patients are admitted only the evening or day before surgery, but sometimes patients have complicating illnesses. They may need to be admitted for optimal control of those problems several days preoperatively.

♦ 3   **Are there any special preoperative instructions that need to be followed, and could I carry these out at home?**

Some surgical procedures require special preparations, e.g., a special diet for several days before bowel surgery.

Often these are carried out in the hospital, but well-motivated patients may be able to manage most special instructions at home. This way they can decrease the required preoperative in-hospital time and decrease costs considerably.

◆ 4   Will you see me in the hospital before surgery?

Your internist will not be your surgeon in nearly all cases. Establish the lines of communication before you arrive at the hospital, so you will know what participation your internist will have in your care both preoperatively and postoperatively.

◆ 5   What are the usual risks of this surgery?

You will have to sign an informed consent form for surgery, which states that you have been told about and understand the risks of the procedure. So make sure you do understand. You may find some things on the list that you had not anticipated and wish to discuss further. Better to do this before a problem occurs.

◆ 6   Do I have any increased risk of surgery because of my particular medical problems?

Any number of medical problems can change the usual risk of surgery and make it a much more serious undertaking. Do you have any of these factors present?

◆ 7   Am I at increased risk for postoperative complications?

Postoperative complications often involve the lungs and incision site, and chances of problems may be increased by underlying lung or heart disease, obesity, drugs you are taking, and a number of other things.

◆ 8   Is there anything I can do now to reduce my risks at surgery?

Patients often can decrease their operative risk even if they have only a short time to make changes. These changes might include stopping smoking, losing weight, or beginning an exercise program.

C H A P T E R T E N

♦

COPING
WITH
ILLNESS:
IS HELP
AVAILABLE?

♦

Many illnesses in adults are chronic or long-term and reflect a gradual deterioration or malfunction of part of the body. For most persons who suffer from these diseases, treatment does not cure the problem. Rather it relieves the symptoms or, at best, slows or stops the progression of disease. Thus, many people will experience increasing disability from illness. These illnesses inevitably influence family, work, and social relationships in insidious and unexpected ways.

Knowing a good deal about your illness, the tests you may undergo, what you can expect during hospitalizations, and how to handle medications will make you feel more comfortable dealing with the disease and the accompanying restrictions on your life. However, coping with the emotional and social aspects of your illness—which may have more impact on your life than the disease itself—often is much more difficult. Furthermore, this inescapable part of the illness is usually the least dealt with by physicians and an area about which they may have little information and few resources.

How can the "nonmedical" ramifications of a disease gain so much importance?

Consider, for example, the 50-year-old man who has been the family breadwinner and is becoming progressively more limited by his emphysema. He finally has to quit his job as a construction foreman, and his wife has to go to work as a secretary. As this happens the man gradually loses his position of power in the family, and family members go to his wife for financial and other important decisions—at the same time as his self-esteem is undermined by inability to work. Suddenly, the family finds its interrelationships strained and its integrity in a crisis. Meanwhile, his drinking buddies seem to be calling less and less because his shortness of breath makes them feel uncomfortable, and he just can't seem to keep up with them anymore. He spends most of the day now sitting in front of the television, drinking alone.

Yes, help is available. In this chapter, I will discuss some issues that arise in many illnesses and ways to plan for or deal with them before a crisis ensues. Many agencies and other sources of information now exist.

These sources of information will be discussed, including organizations dealing with specific illnesses which patients and families can contact.

Patients should not try to or be expected to deal with an illness by themselves. If family members are told and kept informed about a patient's illness, several potential crises can be avoided.

First, the person who is ill needs the compassion and support of family members simply to cope with the physical realities and limitations of the disease. These, of course, are more important in some situations than in others. A patient with paralysis from a stroke will require help with rehabilitation; a patient with kidney disease may need help in adhering to a special and rather strict diet. Many illnesses cause easy fatigue and weakness, which limit the activities the patient can engage in; his family needs to be cognizant and tolerant of this.

Second, the *family* needs to have information about an illness to allow them to plan and prepare for the future. They must also be realistic. What this may entail will vary widely from one situation to another. A young businessman with cancer who has a tumor that is unresponsive to therapy needs to talk to his family about his impending death, how to secure his children's future, his will. Before he can do this, the family needs to be aware of and face the fact that the patient's therapy has failed. Another young construction worker with retinitis pigmentosa who will eventually lose his eyesight may wish to learn some occupation in which he could function with blindness. His wife, who has not been working, may wish to change her plans and prepare herself for a career. To make those decisions, the family must be told of (and must face) the likelihood of the patient's blindness. Preparing in advance could avoid many anxious situations and the downward plunge to welfare of many unfortunate families.

Third, prior knowledge by the family of the emotional stresses that are likely to occur when a family member is ill will help to strengthen rather than disrupt family ties and relationships. These stresses

include, among other things, depression, disappoint-
ment in unfulfilled dreams, loss of self-esteem, possible loss of material wealth, and isolation from
family and friends. Often, early input by health workers and social workers (especially those trained in psychiatry and psychology) can abort potential crises by
supporting a family and pointing out coping mechanisms.

Finally, unexpected complications or sudden flare-
ups of illness can disrupt planned family gatherings,
ceremonies, vacations, and other events. If family
members aren't aware of such possibilities, they are
likely to covertly blame the patient for spoiling the
event, become resentful, feel guilty about these feelings, and a breakdown in communication may occur.
Needless to say, prior knowledge of such possibilities
will not eliminate this type of feeling altogether, since
there is inevitably disruption of family life, but it will
certainly lessen the impact.

Since it is so important to get more general knowledge and help in dealing with illness, I will now focus
on where this help comes from. Your basic understanding of the disease should come from your doctor with
supplementation as I will describe. I have given a number of other sources that will address the total illness—
that is, both the specific physical problems and the
impact of disease on the rest of your life.

ASSOCIATIONS DEALING WITH PARTICULAR ILLNESSES

Probably the best source of information for you is
an association whose purpose is to gain and dissemi-
nate knowledge about your particular illness. Many
common and uncommon illnesses or dramatic illnesses have associations formed by sufferers, families
of sufferers, and other interested persons. If the illness
you have does not have a specific association formed
to deal with it, it will frequently be encompassed by a
more general association that deals with all the diseases, say, relating to an organ system. Diabetes mellitus has its own association, but patients suffering from

coronary artery disease would contact the American
Heart Association or the Canadian Heart Foundation
for information. Patients with artificial heart valves
would also contact either of these associations.

These organizations provide many valuable services. They usually have available printed material
about your disease. Probably more important, they
are familiar with medical, social, and family problems
that are unique to the disease. Often, you can talk to
someone who has had your same problems and has
arrived at some solution. The association will have
names of persons with the disease whom you can contact if you wish. Counseling may also be available. Education and rehabilitation programs may be available
through the association. Fund raising for research into
the illness is often a major activity, and you can become
active in doing this if you wish. The association will
be familiar with the latest approaches to treatment
and experimental approaches to treatment. Ongoing
research projects in which you may wish to participate
are often known to and even financed by these associations. Finally, if you are particularly needy, funds may
be available for various problems related to your illness
or the association may be aware of other funding
sources that are available.

Many associations have educational cassettes, possibly video cassettes, speakers' bureaus, and a variety
of other services that are geared toward patients with
a particular illness. If applicable, they will often be
able to refer you to sources of appropriate appliances,
prostheses, or other devices to aid in the management
of your illness.

How Do You Find Out About These Associations?

Of course, you can ask your doctor. However, it may
be simpler if you live in a moderate to large city to go
to the White Pages of the telephone directory and look
up the illness you have. In more remote areas, this is
difficult, since fewer organizations have small local
chapters. Some organizations dealing with common
illnesses are listed in the appendix.

B O O K S T O R E S

With increasing interest in and desire by people to understand their body and health problems, a number of informative books have been written which give information about a variety of illnesses, drugs, drug interactions, and therapies. Many books about preventive medicine are also available in the health section of bookstores. If you can't find anything about your illness on the shelves, ask the salesperson to check for any books in print. Any books in print can be specially ordered for you.

L I B R A R I E S

Most libraries have good collections of books about health, preventive medicine, and a number of individual illnesses. Some larger libraries have cassettes and cassette-slide programs with information about various health concerns. You may wish to visit a library and look through the books about your illness; then buy the best or most useful one at your bookstore.

D R U G   C O M P A N Y   P U B L I C A T I O N S

Individual drug companies often specialize in drugs for certain types of illnesses. Many of these companies prepare excellent short booklets or pamphlets giving very useful information about etiology of and proper treatment of your illness. Almost always these booklets are free; your doctor or pharmacy may have a supply. If not, you can get the drug company address from your doctor or pharmacy and write to their public relations department requesting information about your illness. Remember, however, that when you get information from drug companies, you are likely to get a bit of advertising of their product as well.

D O C T O R   O R   O T H E R   H E A L T H   C A R E   W O R K E R S

Your doctor, particularly if he specializes in your type of problem, may well have books, pamphlets, or other information for you. These come from drug companies, medical associations, and any of a number of other sources. If he does not have information, he should be able to put you in touch with local resources where you can get help. Sometimes, if your doctor has other patients with the same illness, and these patients are willing, he may be able to arrange for you to contact them. It is often a great help just to be able to contact someone with similar problems. You will probably have contact with a variety of other health care workers during the course of your illness. Nurses, social workers, nutritionists, and other specialists may all have information for you. If your coping problems are more serious, the doctor should be able to refer you to persons trained in helping people cope with the stresses of illness. These might be nurse practitioners trained in psychology or psychiatry, psychologists, or psychiatrists. Your doctor will probably have worked with one or a few of these specialists before and be able to recommend someone who best fills your needs.

H O S P I T A L S

Check with the patient education department of your local hospital. Anything from written materials to a series of classes may be located there, depending on the site of the hospital and local resources. Some hospitals have extensive libraries of information for patients and families. Rehabilitation facilities, out-of-hospital visiting services, or homemaking resources may be available. There may also be a physiotherapy department and a prosthetics department.

G O V E R N M E N T   R E S O U R C E S

Government resources may be available to you if you are disabled and need the assistance of visiting nurses, homemakers, or others. You need to call your county or local federal government offices (Department of Health and Human Services) to find out about eligibility for these programs. In addition, the federal government or the National Institutes of Health have a number of publications available about preventive health care. Social workers may also be able to help with sources of financial aid, improved housing, or whatever your needs are. Public health services are available for some illnesses.

VETERANS' HOSPITALS

If you are a veteran and qualify for care in these facilities, a variety of educational materials and rehabilitation services are usually available. Teaching programs often include classes for diabetics and patients with high blood pressure, heart disease, chronic lung disease, and alcoholism.

MEDICAL ASSOCIATIONS

Though local medical associations are usually associations of doctors, some have educational arms that produce materials for patients. A series of nearly one hundred pamphlets about drug interactions and side effects is published, for example, by the American Medical Association (see Chapter 4 on medications for the address to obtain these). Another prestigious organization of internists, the American College of Physicians, has a program called Health Scope which makes available to schools and other organizations a series of video cassettes and movies about common problems.

HOSPITAL SUPPLY STORES

Often a simple device, like an attachment to help you get in and out of the bathtub, will greatly simplify problems of daily care. Many helpful devices are available to the public through hospital supply stores which you can find by looking in the Yellow Pages. You may not even be aware of what is available, so a call or visit to one of these stores might be worthwhile just to see what they have.

CHAPTER ELEVEN

◆

VOCABULARY

◆

One of the most intimidating places to be is a room full of people who are speaking a foreign language you don't understand. It can be uncomfortable to be in such a situation even when you are an anonymous face in the crowd; but if you are the subject of discussion in these circumstances, feelings of uneasiness might easily turn to fear and anger. Many people have found themselves feeling this way in their doctor's office.

Why? "Medicalese" is one name given to the language doctors or other health professionals use in talking to each other about medical matters. This often sounds like a foreign language to the patient because many of the words are unfamiliar. The use of these terms, despite the feeling of some patients, allows doctors to efficiently and precisely describe locations of illnesses, patient conditions, cause of illness, etc.

The unfamiliar terms that doctors use are almost always from Latin or Greek roots, two or more of which are combined into single words to describe the abnormality that is presumed present plus its appropriate anatomic location. In fact, the language of "medicalese" is very logical and, if you know a few of the roots, very easy to understand. The purpose of this chapter is to help you understand some of the *common* words that may be used in describing your illness and show you how to break words down into their components, which will enable you to figure out the meaning. Also, one section on medication-related terms and another section on test-and-procedure-related terms are included. These words are often not so easy to dissect and understand.

A ◆ WORDS RELATING TO ILLNESS

The first set of roots that are often a part of medical words are those that describe various organs, parts of organs, organ systems, or occasionally areas of the body. Sometimes, one organ has both a Greek and Latin term used, and where this is so, I will include both. This list is not all inclusive but does include most of the commonly used roots. Following the list is an example of how to use the roots to understand unfamiliar terms.

Root Words for Organs / Parts of Organs / Organ Systems / Body Areas

ABDOMINO ◆ Refers to trunk of body below diaphragm usually excluding pelvic organs like uterus, ovaries.

ADENO ◆ Refers to any glands.

ADRENO ◆ Refers to adrenal gland.

ALVEOLI ◆ Saclike structures; most often used to refer to air sacs in lung.

ANGIO ◆ Refers to blood or lymph vessels.

ARTERIO ◆ Refers to arteries.

ARTHRO ◆ Refers to joints.

ATRIO ◆ Chamber or cavity connected to other chambers; refers usually to two upper chambers of heart.

AUDIO ◆ Refers to hearing.

AURI ◆ Refers to ear.

BRONCHO ◆ Refers to airways in lung.

BURS ◆ Refers to small cushioning sacs near joints.

CARDIO ◆ Refers to heart.

CECO ◆ Refers to area of large bowel that joins to small bowel.

CEPHALO ◆ Refers to head.

CERVIC ◆ Can refer to either to neck or to neck of uterus.

CHOLE ◆ Refers to bile.

CHOLECYST ◆ Refers to gallbladder.

CHONDRO ◆ Refers to cartilage.

COLO ◆ Refers to large bowel.

COLPO ◆ Refers to vagina.

COSTO ◆ Refers to ribs.

CYST ◆ Refers to bladder but can be used as a word itself to describe abnormal sac containing gas, fluid, or solid material.

DACRYO ◆ Refers to tears.

DERMO ◆ Refers to skin.

DESMO ◆ Refers to ligament.

DUODENO ◆ Refers to upper part of small bowel.

ENCEPHALO ◆ Refers to brain.

ENDOCRINO ♦ Refers to glands that release internal secretions.

ENTERO ♦ Refers to intestines.

EPIDERMO ♦ Refers to outer skin.

ESOPHAGO ♦ Refers to esophagus, food pipe between mouth and stomach.

GASTRO ♦ Refers to stomach.

GINGIVO ♦ Refers to gums.

GLOSSO ♦ Refers to tongue.

GNATHO ♦ Refers to jaw.

HEMATO ♦ Refers to blood; types of blood cells include white cells and red cells.

HEPATO ♦ Refers to liver.

HYPHOPHYS ♦ Refers to pituitary gland.

HYSTERO ♦ Refers to uterus.

ILEO ♦ Refers to ileum (lower part of small bowel)

ILIO ♦ Refers to ilium (part of pelvic bones)

INTEGUMENT ♦ Skin or body covering.

ISCHIO ♦ Refers to ischium (part of pelvic bones).

JEJUNO ♦ Refers to jejunum (middle part of small bowel).

KERATO ♦ Usually refers to cornea of eye.

LABIO ♦ Refers to lips.

LAPARO ♦ Refers to abdomen.

LARYNGO ♦ Refers to larynx (vocal cords or "voice box").

LEIOMYO ♦ Refers to smooth muscle.

LIPO ♦ Refers to fat or lipid.

LYMPHO ♦ Refers to lymph.

MAMMO ♦ Refers to breasts.

MASTO ♦ Refers to breasts.

MENINGO ♦ Refers to meninges (membranes covering brain and spinal cord).

MUSCULO ♦ Refers to muscle.

MYELO ♦ Refers to bone marrow or the myelin (lining sheath of nerve fibers).

MYO ♦ Refers to muscle.

MYRINGO ♦ Refers to eardrum.

NASO ♦ Refers to nose.

NEPHRO ♦ Refers to kidney.

NEURO ♦ Refers to nerves.

OCULO ♦ Refers to eye.

ODONTO ◆ Refers to teeth.

OMENTO ◆ Refers to omentum (fatty tissue covering abdominal contents.)

OMO ◆ Refers to shoulder.

OMPHALO ◆ Refers to umbilicus.

OOPHORO ◆ Refers to ovary.

OPHTHALMO ◆ Refers to eye.

ORCHIO ◆ Refers to testes.

ORO ◆ Refers to mouth.

OSTEO ◆ Refers to bone.

OVARIO ◆ Refers to ovaries.

OTO ◆ Refers to ear.

PANCREATO ◆ Refers to pancreas (gland secreting digestive enzymes, insulin, and other substances into gut).

PEDO ◆ Refers to feet or child.

PELVI ◆ Refers to pelvis

PERICARDIO ◆ Refers to pericardium (membrane sac around heart).

PERITONEO ◆ Refers to peritoneum (membrane sac lining abdominal cavity).

PHARYNGO ◆ Refers to pharynx (throat).

PHLEBO ◆ Refers to vein.

PHRENO ◆ Refers to diaphragm; can also refer to mind.

PLEURO ◆ Refers to pleura (membrane sac covering lungs).

PNEUMO ◆ Refers to lungs, air, breathing, or occasionally pneumonia.

PODO ◆ Refers to feet.

PROCTO ◆ Refers to anus or rectum (lower part and opening of large bowel).

PROSTATO ◆ Refers to prostate gland.

PROSOPO ◆ Refers to face.

PUBO ◆ Refers to pubis.

PULMO ◆ Refers to lung.

PYELO ◆ Refers to pelvis but usually means a part of the kidney called the kidney pelvis.

PYGO ◆ Refers to buttocks.

RECTO ◆ Refers to rectum.

RENO ◆ Refers to kidney.

RETINO ◆ Refers to retina of eye.

RHABDOMYO ◆ Refers to skeletal muscles.

RHEUMA ◆ Refers to conditions with pain referable

to joints or other parts of musculoskeletal system.

RHINO ♦ Refers to nose.

SACRO ♦ Refers to sacrum (lower backbone).

SALPINGO ♦ Refers to tube, usually fallopian tubes of female genitalia.

SARCO ♦ Refers to muscular substance or a resemblance to flesh.

SCAPULO ♦ Refers to scapula (shoulder blades).

SCLERO ♦ Refers to sclera (white of eye); but also used to mean hardness as in scleroderma, a term meaning hard skin.

SERO ♦ Refers to serum (liquid part of blood).

SIALO ♦ Refers to salivary glands.

SINU; SINO ♦ Refer to sinus, which is a passage for blood or lymph, but sinus commonly used to refer to hollows in the bones of the head surrounding nose or in lower forehead.

SOMATO ♦ Refers to body.

SPINO ♦ Refers to spine or vertebral bones.

SPLANCHNO ♦ Refers to internal organs or viscera.

SPLENO ♦ Refers to spleen (organ composed of lymph tissue which acts as blood filter).

SPONDYLO ♦ Refers to vertebral bones.

STERNO ♦ Refers to sternum or breastbone.

STETHO ♦ Refers to chest.

STOMATO ♦ Refers to mouth.

SYNDESMO ♦ Refers to ligament.

SYNOVIO ♦ Refers to membrane and oils and other elements which line joints and serve as a lubricant cushion.

TALO ♦ Refers to ankle.

TENDO ♦ Refers to tendon.

TENO ♦ Refers to tendon.

THORACO ♦ Refers to chest.

THROMBO ♦ Refers to blood clot.

THYMO ♦ Refers to thymus gland (a gland in the neck which is necessary for normal development of the immune system).

THYRO ♦ Refers to thyroid gland.

TIBIO ♦ Refers to tibia, a bone of the lower leg.

TRACHEO ♦ Refers to trachea, name of airway entering lung until it branches into bronchi.

TRICHO ♦ Refers to hair.

TUBO ♦ Refers to tube, most often fallopian tubes of female genitalia or eustacian tubes of inner ear.

URETERO ♦ Refers to ureter, tube leading from kidney to bladder.

URETHRO ♦ Refers to urethra, tube draining bladder.

URO ♦ Refers to urine.

UTERO ♦ Refers to uterus.

UVEO ♦ Refers to tissues of eye.

UVULO ♦ Refers to uvula

VAGINO ♦ Refers to vagina.

VASCULO ♦ Refers to blood vessels.

VASO ♦ Refers to blood vessels.

VENO ♦ Refers to veins.

VENTRICULO ♦ Refers either to larger chambers of heart or to fluid-containing spaces in brain.

VERTEBRO ♦ Refers to vertebrae (bones of spine).

VESICO ♦ Refers to urinary bladder.

VESTIBULO ♦ Refers to inner portions of ear.

XIPHO ♦ Refers to bottom end of breastbone (xiphoid).

A root denoting an organ, part of organ, or other anatomical part of the body will often be connected to one or more other roots (as either prefixes or suffixes) which describe the disease process(es) in that organ, other changes in the organ (not necessarily disease), or a manipulation that involves the "root" anatomy. I have divided these descriptive terms into prefixes and suffixes.

P R E F I X E S

a-   without
ab-   away from
acro-   extremity, tip
ad-   toward
aden-   gland
adip-   fatty
alge-, algo-, algesi-   pain
allo-   other
an-   without
aniso-   dissmilar
antero-   anterior
anti-   against

apo- separated from
auto- self
baso- toward the base
bi- twice
brachy- short
brady- slow
carci- type of cancer
cata- down
cauda- tail or toward tail
ceno- shared in common
centro- center
chemo- chemistry
cirrh- tawny or yellow (relating to liver)
cyano- blue
cyto- cell
de- negative or away from
di- two
dis- take apart
dista- away from
dorsi- posterior or near back surface
dys- bad or difficult
ec- out of; away from
ecto- outside
em- in
en- in
endo- within
epi- upon
erythr- red
eso- within
eu- good; well
ex- out of; away from
exo- exterior, external
ferri- iron
fibrino- related to blood clot
fibro- fiber (scar tissue)
galact- milk
gero-, geron- old age
gluco- sugar
glyc- sugar
gyne- woman
hemi- half
hetero- other or different
hidr- sweat

histio- tissue
histo- tissue
holo- whole
homeo- same or alike
homo- same or alike
hyal- glassy
hydro- water
hyper- excessive
hypo- deficiency; beneath something else (location)
iatro- denotes relation to physicians, medicine,
    treatment
ichthy- fishlike
idio- one's own; used to denote cause unknown
immuno- relating to immunity
in- within; negative
iodo- iodine
iso- equal; like
karyo- nucleus
kerato- horny tissue
kinesi- related to motion
lacri- tear
lacti- milk
latero- to one side or relating to the side
leuk-, leuc- white
litho- stone; calcification
lyo- to dissolve
lys- to dissolve
macro- large, long
meato- opening or passage
media- middle; toward the center
medullo- center
mega-, megalo- oversize
melan- black; dark
membrano- referring to a membrane
meso- middle or near
meta- after; behind; subsequent to; sometimes
    refers to a transformation or joint action
micro- smallness
mono- single
muci-, muco- mucous
multi- many
myco-, myceto- fungus
myxo- mucous

necro- death
neo- new
noso- refers to disease; in nosocomial, means hospital
nucleo- nucleus
occipito- back of head
ochro- yellow
odont- teeth
oligo- few or a little
onco- tumor
onycho- nail
organo- denoting an organ
ortho- proper order, straight; normal
oxy- oxygen
pachy- thick
pan- all
papulo- small elevation on skin
para- departure from normal, alongside; near
path- disease
pedi- child
peri- around; about
pero- malformed
phaco-, phako- lens-shaped
phago- eating; devouring
phyco- seaweed
physio- physical
phyto- plants
platy- flat
pleo- more or many
poikilo- irregular; varied
poly- many
poro- passage
postero- posterior
pro- forward
pseudo- resemblance, often deceptive
psycho- mind
py-, pyo- pus
pyg- buttocks
pyk-, pykno- thick, dense, compact
quadri- four
radio- radiation
reticulo- network (of cells)
retro- behind

rhizo- root
rubri- red
sacchar- sugar
sapro- rotten, decayed
sarco- muscle or resemblance to flesh
schizo- split
scler- hardness
semi- one half or partly
septic- presence of pus-forming organisms
septo- septum
sero- serum
sialo- saliva
sicc- dry
sidero- iron
spheno- wedge-shaped
sphero- sphere
sphygm- pulse
sporo- seed
squam- scale (upper skin)
stearo- fat
steato- fat
stereo- three-dimensional
stetho- chest
sub- beneath; less than normal
super- above the part indicated, excess
supra- above the part indicated
sympath- relates to part of the nervous system
tachy- rapid
tel-, telo- distance; end
temporo- denotes temples at sides of head
terato- misshapen; abnormal parts
tetra- four
thermo- heat
thrombo- blood clot
toco- childbirth
tomo- cutting (a section)
toxo-, toxico- poison
trans- through, beyond
traum- wound; injury
tri- three
tropho- food; nutrition
ultra- excess; beyond
uni- one; single

ure-, ureo-, uro,- urea or urine
vari- dilated vein
ventro- anterior
vesiculo- blister
vestibulo- small space at the entrance (to something)
xantho- yellow
xeno- strange; foreign
xero- dry
zygo- yolk; joining

Suffixes

-algesia sense of pain
-algia pain; painful condition
-arthria to articulate
-asthenia weakness
-atric relating to medicine, healing
-cele swelling or hernia
-centesis puncture (usually to remove fluid)
-chezia to go to stool
-chrome color
-clasis, -clastic broken
-cyte cell
-dactyly finger or toe
-desis bind together
-dynia pain
-ectasia, -ectasis dilation or expansion
-ectomy removal of an anatomical structure
-edema swelling
-emesis vomiting
-ema, -emia blood
-enclesis shut in
-esia, -esis condition, action, process
-genic, -genous, -genesis producing or forming
-gnosia, -gnosis knowledge
-gram a recording
-graphy to record function
-ia condition
-iasis condition
-ites, -itis inflammation
-kinesia, -kinesis movement
-lateral to the side

-lithic relating to stone, calcification
-lithiasis stone(s)
-lysis destruction; subsiding of symptoms
-malacia softness
-megaly large
-morphic form; shape
-necrosis death (with implied degeneration)
-oid resembling
-olisthesis falling or slipping
-ology science of
-oma tumor
-ose full of
-osis process; condition, state
-ostomy an artificial opening; surgery in which
    opening is made between two hollow organs, or
    hollow organ and abdominal wall
-osus full of
-otomy cutting operation
-palsy partial paralysis
-paresis partial paralysis
-pathy disease
-penia deficiency
-pexy fix
-phage, -phagia, -phagy eating; devouring
-phasia speech
-philia, -phil, -philic affinity or craving for
-phobia, -phobic morbid dread or fear
-phonia voice
-phoria a carrying; motion
-phyma tumor
-plasia formation
-plasty molding or shaping (usually as result of
    surgery)
-plegia paralysis
-pnea breath, respiration
-poietic, -poiesis production
-ptosis falling; downward displacement of organ
-ptysis spitting
-rrhagia excessive or unusual discharge
-rrhapy surgical suturing; seam
-rrhea flowing or flux
-rrhexis rupture
-rrhiza root

-schisis   clearing
-sclerosis   harding
-scopy   activity involving an instrument for viewing
-static, -stasis   standing still
-staxis   to fall in drops
-stoma, -stomia   mouth; opening
-syndesis   a binding
-tasis   stretching
-taxis   orderly arrangement
-tomy   cutting operation
-tonic   strength, tone, tension
-tony   tone, tension
-tresia, -tresis   a hole
-trophic, -tropia   a turning toward, affinity for
-trophy   food, nutrition
-uretic   denotes urine
-uria   denotes urine

The following are some examples of how roots, prefixes, and suffixes are combined to succinctly describe diseases, conditions, and other medical situations.

If you have hematuria, you have blood in your urine.
    BLOOD   URINE

If you have had a laparotomy with a cholecyst-
                  ABDOMEN CUTTING   GALLBLADDER
                          OPERATION

ectomy and colectomy with colostomy, you have had
REMOVAL   COLON REMOVAL   COLON OPENING
                                TO ABDOMINAL
                                WALL

abdominal surgery with removal of the gallbladder
and part of the colon and an opening has been made
from the colon to the abdominal wall.

You wake up feeling lousy. You have myalgias,
                                    MUSCLE PAIN

arthralgias, and pleurodynia. You report to an emer-
JOINT   PAIN   MEMBRANE PAIN
                   COVERING
                   LUNG

gency room where you are found to be euthermic,

NORMAL TEMPERATURE
(GOOD)

but a sample of your blood obtained by venipuncture

VEIN

reveals a mild leukopenia, with a relative lymphocyt-

WHITE DEFICIENCY
CELL

LYMPH CELL

osis. That is, you have muscle aches, joint pains, and

STATE

chest pain. At the emergency room you do not have a fever, but your blood shows a slightly decreased white blood count, but with a large number of lymphocytes.

B ♦ WORDS USED WITH MEDICATIONS

adjuvant—Means to give aid to. (1) In cancer, it means therapy that is sometimes used in conjunction with surgery, even when no obvious tumor remains, because of improvement in cure rates. (2) Can also mean substances added to a drug which affects action in a predictable way.

ampule—Sealed container (usually glass) containing medication in solution or powder to be reconstituted with fluid.

ante—Before.

b.i.d.—(bis in die) Twice a day (not necessarily 12 hours apart).

biofeedback—Technique allowing person to gain voluntary control over a usually involuntary action.

blood level—Refers to amount of drug in the blood at a specific time.

capsule—Powdered drug or drug in small beads contained in a gelatin shell.

consolidation—Used in cancer drug therapy. Refers to courses of therapy after the initial phase meant to ensure either cure or prolonged disease-free interval.

contraindication—An absolute reason not to take a certain drug.

courses—Usually used in cancer therapy. Refers to a given pattern of drug administration. Each repitition of the pattern is called a course: e.g., drug may be given for five days with a three-week rest period. Each five-day administration is a course.

diurnal—Rhythm, repeating once each 24 hours. Usually refers to daily variations of internal hormone levels.

diuretic—Causes excretion of urine.

divided doses—When a certain total dose of a drug is required per day, rather than giving it all at one time, it will be given in several divided doses over the day to maximize effectiveness or ease of taking it.

dosing interval—Number of hours between doses.

double strength—Double usual dose of drug contained in one pill, capsule, etc.

DS—Double strength

elixir—A sweetened liquid, often with alcohol base, used as vehicle for carrying medicines.

enteric coated—Drug has coating which will not dissolve in acid environment of stomach but will dissolve in alkaline environment of intestine.

generic—General; used to refer to chemical name, rather than drug company brand name, of a drug. Drugs available generically may be less expensive than those formulated and sold through a drug company.

gm—Gram.

gr—(Granum) Grain; 1 grain = 65 milligrams.

gt, gh—(gutta, guttae) Drop, drops.

half-life—Time taken for one half of administered radioactive substance to be lost through biological process. Also used to refer to time taken for one half of drug to be converted to inactive compound or eliminated from body.

H.S.—(Hora Somni) Just before sleep.

IM—Intramuscular; mode of giving drug by syringe and needle in muscle.

induction—Used to refer to the phase of cancer drug therapy when an attempt is made to rid the patient of obvious cancer; intensive initial drug therapy, often followed by consolidation phase if successful. Also, initial drug(s) given to render a person unconscious (anesthetized) prior to surgery.

intradermal—In the skin.

IV—Intravenous; mode of giving drug by needle into vein.

IV piggyback—Drug mixed in small bag of fluid and fed into a needle port on an existing intravenous line.

IV push—Method of injecting medication full strength directly into vein.

loading dose—Extra amount of drug given as a first dose to rapidly establish a desired level in the blood.

maintenance dose—Amount of drug needed per dosing interval to maintain a desired amount in the blood.

mg—Milligram.

O.D.—(oculo dextro) In the right eye.

o.d.—(omni die) Every day.

O.S.—(oculo sinistro) In the left eye.

O.U.—(oculo utra) In each eye.

palliative—Meant only to lessen symptoms, not to cure.

p.c.—(post cibum) After meals.

peak level—Highest level (largest amount) of drug.

p.o.—(per os) By mouth.

postlevel—Refers to amount of drug in the blood shortly after a dose is given.

prelevel—Refers to amount of a drug in the blood shortly before a dose is given.

p.r.n.—(pro re nata) As occasion rises. Usually written, e.g., "every 4 hours p.r.n." It means you may take it every 4 hours if you need it, but not more often.

prophylactic—Preventive; refers to drug given to prevent development of symptom or disease.

pulse—Refers to method of giving a drug in which a few large doses are given, rather than smaller, more chronically administered doses.

q.d.—(quaque die) Each day.

q __ h—(quaque horae) Every __ hours.

q.s.—(quantum sufficit) Enough.

q.i.d.—(quater in die) Four times a day.

s.c.—(subcutaneous) Under the skin.

side effect—Symptom, organ malfunction or other change caused by a drug.

sig.—(signa) Label.

slow release—Drug is formulated to be released slowly over a given period of time, usually 8 to 12 hours.

ss.—(semis) One half.

stat—(statim) Immediately.

suppository—A small solid body containing medication and meant to be placed in a body orifice other than the mouth. Melts and releases medication at body temperature.

tablet—Powdered drug pressed into formed pill without coating.

teratogenic—Causes birth defects.

t.i.d.—(ter in die) Three times a day.

topical—Drug placed on surface of body.

toxic level—Amounts of drug associated with potentially harmful or irreversible side effects.

trough level—The least amount of drug in the blood between doses, usually just before a dose is given.

unit dose—Refers to individual packaging of doses of drug to decrease possibility of medication errors, especially overdosing.

C ◆ WORDS USED WITH PROCEDURES AND TESTS

Please refer to Chapter Five for a brief description of most types of tests. Included below are some general terms you may encounter when preparing for or undergoing tests.

AP—Anterior-posterior: opposite of usual way a chest x-ray is taken; refers to x-rays taken by portable equipment.

aspirate—Remove with a needle and syringe.

barium studies—Refers to x-rays of hollow viscera taken after patient has either swallowed or been given enema of radiopaque barium to better outline the structures.

bilateral—When study or condition involves organ system in which there is pair of organs, e.g., means both of the organs are involved or studied.

biopsy—Remove a small piece of tissue for diagnostic reasons.

bowel prep—Refers to a series of manipulations (ranging from diet changes to laxatives to enemas) to prepare for bowel studies.

camera—Refers to scanner in nuclear studies which records radioactivity.

cannulate—Refers to act of placing a catheter in a blood or lymph vessel.

C-arm—Refers to type of x-ray machine which can be rotated around the patient to take x-rays at different angles.

cassette—Refers to the device containing film on x-ray equipment.

catheter—Hollow, flexible, usually plastic tube to be placed in body orifice or vessel for purpose of carrying out a study or administering substances.

closed biopsy—Piece of tissue is taken through skin without direct visualization of the organ biopsied.

complication—Adverse side effect resulting from a test or procedure. May or may not have lasting effect on patient.

diagnosis—Exact definition of a disease process.

distal—Refers to part of organ or limb farthest from center of body.

dye study—Any procedure in which a radiopaque dye is injected into a body space in order to better outline structures.

ECG (or EKG) monitor—Placing of electrodes on chest to monitor heartbeat throughout procedure. (Usually visible on overhead screen.)

end-diastolic pressure—Pressure in left heart just before a beat (contraction).

end-systolic pressure—Pressure in left heart just at the end of a beat (contraction).

endobronchial—Within the airway.

endoscope—Device to look inside body organs via body orifices (see next definition).

fiberoptic scope—Any of several devices designed for evaluation of various organ systems. Consists of bundle of flexible plastic fibers to the far end, having a plastic cover and fitted with a series of lenses. Portions of the body, e.g., stomach, remote from the viewer (outside the body), can be visualized by images reflected back through the scope.

films—Refers to x-rays.

flat plate—Refers to x-ray of abdomen taken with patient lying down.

fluoroscopy—Refers to a type of x-ray machine that can be used like a movie camera in viewing dynamics of the body.

general—Refers to general anesthetic, or anesthesia which renders the patient unconscious for the procedure.

hematoma—Collection of blood outside of vessel but within body.

intraarterial—Within an artery.

intraop—Means during the procedure or operation.

intravenous—Within a vein.

label—Refers to a radioactive particle which, because of its radioactivity, can be traced by a scanner once it is in the body.

lateral—Refers to x-ray taken with side of patient's body facing camera.

local—Refers to local anesthesia, or locally applied drug which renders a small area insensitive to pain.

mucosal—Refers to something involving the surface (mucosa) of the hollow internal organs.

needle biopsy—A type of closed biopsy taken by passage of a hollow needle usually through skin into the organ to be sampled.

NPO—Means nothing by mouth (often for several hours before test).

oblique—Refers to an angled position in which the patient is placed relative to a scanner or x-ray machine to get a better view of a specific area.

open biopsy—The removal of a small piece of an organ, usually at surgery, where the organ is directly visualized.

osmotic diuresis—Excessive urination caused by presence in blood of very "dense" fluid, often the dye used in procedures.

PA—Posterior-anterior; refers to usual way in which a chest x-ray is taken.

percutaneous—Through the skin; many closed biopsies are taken percutaneously.

polyp—mass of tissue projecting out from surface.

postop—Refers to the immediate postoperative (or postprocedure) period; may refer to postoperative orders to be carried out.

preop—Refers to medications given to a patient just before a procedure, usually to mildly sedate the patient.

prep—(preparation) Refers to whatever measures are necessary to ready the patient for the procedure.

pressure dressing—A dressing placed over a site likely to bleed (artery, e.g.), in such a way that pressure is increased in an attempt to stop or prevent bleeding.

pressure monitor—Refers to monitoring of blood pressure or any of several other pressures, usually by catheters in body vessels or spaces during a study. This is usually produced as a tracing on video monitor.

prone—Lying on one's stomach.

proximal—Refers to part of limb or organ closest to center of body.

scanner—Camera used in recording radioactivity during a nuclear scan; also, used to refer to the x-ray machine used in CT scans (see Chapter 5).

submucosal—Beneath the lining layer (mucosa) of the hollow internal organs.

supine—Lying on one's back.

transbronchial—Means through the wall of the airway.

ulcer—Loss of normal covering of tissue with inflammation.

unilateral—When study or condition involves organ system with a pair of organs, e.g., kidneys, means only one of the organs is involved or studied.

upright—Describes x-ray taken with the patient standing.

venous access—Means catheter placement into a vein so that blood can be removed or substances added to the bloodstream.

APPENDIX

The following is a list of organizations that deal with certain types of illness discussed in Chapter 3. Many other groups dealing with other illnesses also exist. These are often listed in the white pages of the telephone book under the name of the disease or organ involved.

1. ARTHRITIS

Arthritis Foundation
1314 Spring St. N.W.
Atlanta, GA 30309
(404) 972-7100

Canadian Arthritis
  Society
250 Bloor St. E.
Suite #420
Toronto, Ontario M4W
  3P2
(416) 967-1414

Lupus Foundation of
  America
11921 Olive Blvd.
St. Louis, MO
(314) 872-9036

Ontario Lupus
  Association
250 Bloor St. E.
Suite #401
Toronto, Ontario M4W
  3P2
(416) 967-1414

2. ASTHMA;
   EMPHYSEMA/
   CHRONIC
   BRONCHITIS

American Lung
  Association
1740 Broadway
New York, NY 10019
(212) 245-8000

Canadian Lung
  Association
75 Albert St.
Suite #908
Ottawa, Ontario K1P
  5E7
(616) 237-1208

3. CANCER

American Cancer
  Society Inc.
90 Park Ave., Second
  Floor
New York, NY 10016
(212) 599-8200

National Cancer
  Institute of Canada
130 Bloor St. W.
Suite #1001
Toronto, Ontario M5S
  2V7
(416) 961-7223

4. CORONARY ARTERY
   DISEASE (OR ANY
   OTHER HEART
   DISEASE)
   American Heart
     Association
   7320 Greenville Ave.
   Dallas, TX 75231
   (214) 750-5300

   Canadian Heart
     Foundation
   1 Nicholas St.
   Suite #1200
   Ottawa, Ontario K1N
     7B7
   (613) 237-4361

5. DIABETES MELLITUS
   American Diabetes
     Assoc. Inc.
   2 Park Ave.
   New York, NY 10017
   (212) 683-1444

   Canadian Diabetes
     Assoc.
   78 Bond St.
   Toronto, Ontario M5B
     2J8
   (416) 362-4440

6. KIDNEY DISEASE
   AND HIGH BLOOD
   PRESSURE
   Kidney Foundation
     (National)
   2 Park Ave.
   Suite #908
   New York, NY 10016
   (212) 889-2210

   Kidney Foundation of
     Canada
   1300 Yonge St.
   Toronto, Ontario M4T
     1X3
   (416) 925-2836

7. LIVER DISEASE
   American Liver
     Foundation
   998 Pompton Ave.
   Cedar Grove, NJ 07009
   (201) 857-2626

   Canadian Liver
     Foundation
   42 Charles St.
   Toronto, Ontario M4Y
     1T4
   (416) 964-1953

8. STROKES
   Stroke Foundation Inc.
   898 Park Ave.
   New York, NY 10021
   (212) 734-3461

   Canadian Heart
     Foundation
   1 Nicholas St.
   Suite #1200
   Ottawa, Ontario K1N
     7B7
   (613) 237-4361

◆

INDEX

◆

Emotional involvement, with doctor, 21–22
Emotional stress, 166–67
Emphysema, 75, 123, 165
  see also Lung disease
Endoscopy, 90, 91, 113, 139
  fiberoptic, 116–17
Environment
  and cancer, 58
  and coronary artery disease, 69–70
  and lung disease, 74–75
Epilepsy, 105
Equipment, for stroke victims, 89
Esophagoscopy, 116
Ethical/moral problem, and changing doctor, 149
Euthermic, 186
Exercise, 44, 163
  and arthritis, 51
  and asthma, 53–54
  for coronary artery disease, 69
Eye complications, 73

Facilities, for cancer, 64–65
Family, 46–47
  and cancer, 58
  and emotional stress, 166–67
Fees, conflicts over, 151
  see also Charges; Financial arrangements; Payment
Fetal malformations, 105
Fetus
  and nuclear scans, 115
  and x-rays, 113–14
Fiberoptic endoscopy, 116–117
Financial arrangements, for hospitalization, 161–162

  see also Charges; Fees; Payment
Fluoroscopic x-rays, 112, 113
Follow-up care, 25, 27, 44
Food, and drugs, 102–3
Full life support, 65

Gallbladder surgery, 43, 143
Gallstones, 128
Gastrointestinal x-rays, 112–13
Gastroscopy, 116, 124
Generic drugs, 104–5
Genetic factors, 39
  and coronary artery disease, 69–70
  see also Heredity
Glucose (sugar), 71
Gout, 52
Government resources, 170–71

Hamartomas, 34
Health care workers, 170
Health insurance, 45
  and diabetes, 74
Health Scope (health program), 171
Heart, 33, 111
  blood vessels to, 65
  medications for, 66–68
  surgery for, 24, 66, 68
Heart attack (myocardial infarction), 66, 100
  complications after, 66
  sexual intercourse without risk of, 69
  and surgery, 68
Heart disease, 60, 67, 72, 83
  and diet, 68–69
  see also Coronary artery disease
Heart failure, 99, 100
Heart Foundation, 90

204 I N D E X

ABOUT THE
AUTHOR

◆

Dr. Janet Maurer is currently practicing in Toronto, Canada, where she is Director of the Respirology (Pulmonary) Clinical Service of the Toronto General Hospital and Assistant Professor of Medicine at the University of Toronto. She is a member of the American College of Physicians, the American College of Chest Physicians, and the American Thoracic Society, and is a Fellow of the Royal College of Physicians & Surgeons of Canada.